Akashic Therapy

Unlock the Secrets of Your Soul

AMANDA ROMANIA

BALBOA
PRESS
A DIVISION OF HAY HOUSE

ISBN: 978-1-4525-3660-6 (sc)
ISBN: 978-1-4525-3661-3 (e)
Library of Congress Control Number: 2011911788

Balboa Press books may be ordered through booksellers or by contacting:
Balboa Press
A Division of Hay House
1663 Liberty Drive
Bloomington, IN 47403
www.balboapress.com
1-(877) 407-4847

Because of the dynamic nature of the Internet, any web addresses or links contained in this book may have changed since publication and may no longer be valid. The views expressed in this work are solely those of the author and do not necessarily reflect the views of the publisher, and the publisher hereby disclaims any responsibility for them.

The author of this book does not dispense medical advice or prescribe the use of any technique as a form of treatment for physical, emotional, or medical problems without the advice of a physician, either directly or indirectly. The intent of the author is only to offer information of a general nature to help you in your quest for emotional and spiritual well-being. In the event you use any of the information in this book for yourself, which is your constitutional right, the author and the publisher assume no responsibility for your actions.

Any people depicted in stock imagery provided by Thinkstock are models, and such images are being used for illustrative purposes only. Certain stock imagery © Thinkstock.

Printed in the United States of America
Balboa Press rev. date: 9/13/2011

For my daughter Scarlett who brought the love and light and husband Stephen who opened the door to a dream.

CONTENTS

Standing in the Vortex Falling
Eyes are all around me Watching
Through the Mist of time I'm gazing
Stepping through the veils that are Lifting
Connecting to my Heart Directly
Seeing myself Now Absolutely
Hearing my Beloved Calling
Manifesting My Reality Totally
Open the Doorway, I'm Ready

—Amanda Romania, 2007

PART ONE

The Invitation

Join Me on the Akashic Journey

Welcome.
- Have you ever had déjà vu?
- Have you felt a strong connection to someone or dislike of a person on first meeting?
- Do you ever have physical symptoms that can't be explained and that come and go for no reason?
- Do you ever connect with a period of history so much, you wish you lived then?
- Are there countries you have no desire to visit, spaces and places you fantasize about, or locations you could never leave?
- Do you feel that inner peace and understanding is only a moment away but still out of your reach?
- Do you want to know more about the soul journey and your divine purpose in life?
- Do you wonder about the karma you carry and how that can affect this and the next soul life?

If you have answered yes to any of these questions, then I am delighted you were guided to my book today. You have taken a step toward listening and opening your heart and soul to finding the next stage on your spiritual quest. May you find the inner bliss, beauty, and balance you have been seeking.

Please allow me to take you on a journey to awaken your inner sanctuary and lift the veils of your deep knowing.

The Akashic records are the database of the universe; we all have a unique file. This file holds the story of your soul, with all the light and dark, negative and positive. It has been my role for many years to guide others through their lives and heal and clear all that does not serve them. I came to see this process as a therapy and in service of the soul's spiritual quest.

Akashic therapy works with a Divine Heart meditation to examine the past, present, life between lives and future lives. These lives are found in your Akashic records. Often defined as a metaphysical concept, it relates to the transcendent or to a reality beyond what is perceptible to the senses.

I have a passion and purpose to support others on their spiritual journey. Using my gifts in this book to engage you with your heart and essence, I will teach you how to understand universal energy and how to apply this to everyday life.

As you move gently through this empowering book, you develop skills to use all your spiritual gifts and senses to find an inner peace and understanding of your spiritual purpose at this time.

You will give a voice to your subconscious like it has never experienced before and a method to bring positive affirmation into your life at a deeper level.

My experience with the Akashic records is extensive over the past decade, having worked with indigenous elders and shamans in the realm of sacred site energy, ritual, and Egyptian initiation. I'll share my stories and knowledge throughout the chapters.

I humbly invite you to open the veils to the mysteries of your Akashic records.

NEW GENERATION LIVING

Every moment, we are creating our reality, like a thread of beads. We add to it constantly with thoughts and actions.

The planets and universe around us are in constant motion, also shifting on all holistic levels. For many, the shift is not about world disaster but about a new paradigm time when we go from *Homo sapiens* to *"Homo luminous"* or enlightened beings. We are evolving as a species on many levels with our own timelines and collective consciousness.

Many have heard the call to action, and it is now their passion to raise awareness and connection to spirit. Many know they have a greater purpose on the planet; they just have limited clarity to focus on a clear intention or direction.

While you connect daily with the external elements of our world, how often do you go inside yourself, to the deep recess, to your core and let your soul speak?

Many of us are afraid—afraid of what we may find, and that is why this Akashic journey is different from others. There is no fear, only enlightenment.

Akashic therapy accesses the information through a heart meditation, talking directly to your source or core soul. I was taught how to use this gift through my many adventures and journeys through the sacred sites of the world. Now the vibration of the planet is changing, its time for me to lift the veils, to share my story and teaching with you.

This book is intended to act as an easy read of stories and examples. This is mixed with a workbook of exercises, to allow you to set intention, work with your heart, call your guides, and visit the areas within your Akashic records for answers to your questions and then create some questions to your answers. It's also layered with the etheric codes and keys that I have used to connect with the other dimensions and search further.

It's a like a treasure map; you just need to trust and follow to where X marks the spot.

So just relax, breathe, and hold this affirmation:

*I am connected to the universe in
energy, heart, and soul.
Time has no limits for me.
I connect to Gaia, who nurtures me.
I reach for the stars that embrace me.
I am ready to see the journey of my soul.
I am safe.
I am love.*

Karma Dharma

Everyone holds Karma in his or her Akashic records. The Karma can be positive or negative. There is no judgment; it simply is the cause and effect that you personally create. Dharma operates with the law of nature and is the balance of life. Clearing Karma rebalances Dharma.

In the past, these cycles of karma were rebalanced in the next life. We are all on the Wheel of Dharma, it seems. During this time, however, I am finding that not only is past-life karma recurring in a person's life but also their current-life karma as well.

Yes, this can be confusing.

This is due to the new levels of consciousness we are reaching. We are moving into a whole new stage of enlightenment.

Now is the time for us to release our karmic baggage with ease and grace. It is this baggage that holds us back.

For many years, I have worked with the ascended masters who guide this cycle of life. When I was starting this book, I asked them what they wished to share with my readers.

MESSAGE FROM THE LORDS
AND LADIES OF KARMA

*Beloved earthbound souls, for many lifetimes, you
have moved forward with your journey of life and
path of evolution, many of you praying for release
from the karma which holds you to this circle of life.*

*We watch and reach out toward you with compassion
and care and in this lifetime have created the
energetic force to release many of you and allow
others to flow with karma clearance in this lifetime.*

*This enables your soul energy to release back into
the universe to join with the next phases and stages
of existence and life.*

*We hold no judgment, only hope and gratitude
in our souls for the paths that you choose and
the messages that you send.*

But in the end, two choices are always clear: fear or love.

*Love and peace will heal the energy streams.
You tangle your path and hold yourself back from the
relationships and purpose you seek. We only wish
to bring joy to your life.*

*Focus forward with joy and happiness, and we
will support and clear the way.*

What Was My Personal Journey?

I personally believe that this is a time of awakening to a new consciousness, and many people ask when I felt I had my clairvoyant sight to see the unknown.

I remember as a child having very strong intuitive skills. I was petite for my age and sometimes vulnerable to bullies. However, I learned quickly how to move though a situation and align myself not with trouble but with a crowd of popular girls. I was not a queen bee, but I was not open prey either. I guess I always felt I had protection around me. I would often know the outcome of a situation. Strong intuition and emotional intelligence developed early on in my life.

Working in retail very successfully for many years opened my life to people of all ages, and during my late twenties, I started to question my life. When I was thirty, I had my daughter, Scarlett. I went from high-flying executive to distraught housemother. As a baby, Scarlett had egg and food allergies, which were not diagnosed until she was a year old. This had meant twelve months of no sleep and a baby who scratched herself until she bled. Panic, pain, shame, and guilt; yes, I carried and wore all of those sad, soul-destroying badges. There had to be another way. My natural motherly instinct kicked in, which kicked a lot of trust in the medical system out. Thankfully, I was referred to a homeopath who, within a month, had rebalanced her system, and I had a magical, delightful child.

I began to investigate well-being and alternative methods further. I began creative manifesting and meditating. My life was clearly turning around. By the time Scarlett was five, I was working in my own business with an amazing team of women.

This allowed me time and resources to travel and explore more of life.

I came across a personal life coach who ran a self-help business workshop. My marriage was coming to an amicable end, and I needed a positive aspect in my life to help me focus forward. And that it did, as it opened up awareness with spirit and the emotions of others.

I remember in one self-help session working with a lady, we had decided to meditate on her mother. While in the space of connection, I felt a heated sensation all the way down my left side and a burning in my chest. When we finished, I turned to the woman and explained this. She began to cry. "My mum has breast cancer," she whispered. "She just had chemotherapy on her left side."

Wow, this was a wakeup to an unknown realm of life. I was totally blown away. We just sat silently for a long time. Then we both cried and said prayers for her family.

After this workshop, I was inspired to detox my life in many ways. My divorce was pending, my business flowing, and my daughter and I were taking care of each other in our little sanctuary home. We had the whole house cleared of old fixtures and fittings and painted cream throughout. Cleansing on all levels. This was an ivory tower.

I decided to then go on a full-body detox cleanse to Portugal—the best and worst choice ever. I never read the small print about how difficult it was to give up caffeine and other delightful toxic foods and drinks. If it had not been for my amazing roommate and newfound soul sister, an American woman who was like a walking angel, I think I would be lost forever. After the first week, I was like a zombie shuffling around in a quilt, having strange dreams and reading angel cards for everyone with scary accuracy. I felt and looked deranged.

At this point, a therapist who was working on the spiritual healing section of the detox took me to her cabin, sat me down with her motherly authority, and placed a pendulum in my hand. "Show me," she said sharply.

I held it by its cord and stretched out my arm. My other hand shook in fear and anticipation.

"It's swinging," I replied. "What does that mean?" I was now terrified as this crystal swung around like it was possessed.

She laughed and gently began to ask questions about my dreams and state of mind. She then leaned forward and whispered, "You're awakening, darling. You're finding your clairvoyant sight." We talked for a little longer about my understanding of the messages I had in my head, the pictures I was seeing in my dreams, which she thought perfectly normal.

I left her and shuffled back to my room, for the first time in months with a feeling of peace of heart and soul that I was not going crazy. As I left, I claimed my power back. I was walking through the orchard and took an orange from a tree. I hid behind a wall and ate the fruit. It was like liquid sunshine, and I found myself in a column of sunlight, both around me and running through me. I felt no guilt in breaking the juice fast. I felt a connection with something more divine. I felt like every tree and flower around me heard and understood. I was never so grateful for that gift of light and love from nature. I went back to my room and cried for four hours. I cried every layer of grief that was in me. And when it was done, I began to plan and think about a new life for my daughter and me.

After the detox, my spiritual growth and path moved very quickly. I returned to the UK and visited my new American sister, who was living at Buckland Hall in Wales. This was the magical place where J.R.R. Tolkien had taken inspiration for the Lord of the Rings stories. For days, we walked in the gardens, and I felt brought back to life by the lush greenery; it was like being in an oxygen chamber. I began to read more oracle cards, and my vision skills improved. I was using my intuition in all aspects of life and for others also.

From Buckland, I received an invitation to visit California and attend a gathering of elders and sacred grandmothers at Big Bear Mountain. Upon meeting them in a hotel foyer at Los Angeles International Airport, there was an instant connection.

Grandma Connie, the Hopi elder, grasped both my hands and stared deep into me.

"You were with us last gathering," she said. "I remember you."

"No, Grandma Connie," I replied quietly, shaking my head.

"Then it was in a time passed by," she said firmly, nodding her head and looking me straight in the eyes.

I assumed this was old-lady talk; however, on reflection, this was a moment of great significance for me and deeply connected to past lives and my soul purpose. I traveled with the sacred grandmothers, and to my surprise, they invited me to live with them in their room. It was a small cabin with eight bunk beds. I was on the top corner, above Grandmother Flordemayo, a Mayan priestess. Of course I had no idea how special, gifted, or amazing these women were.

That was until I opened the door one morning and found a stream of people waiting outside with offerings, gifts, and prayers. My role was simple: help the grandmothers prepare, keep them safe in ceremony, and make cups of tea when the work and ritual was complete. This I did in my pink track suit and sparkle sandals, which I think everyone found rather interesting, as most were in tie-dye and new-age ethnic rainbow clothes with unique tribal jewelry.

I was truly blessed. I was able to see the grandmothers as women first. I listened to their stories about their husbands and children, and their concerns for Mother Earth and how they would pay for their next journey of service. All agreed it was in the hands of spirit and to open and trust.

During this time, I was having regular lucid dreams and remember thinking *I'm here as a witness, an observer, or a record-keeper.* I was taking in information and recording it to report the story at some later time in history.

This trip with the grandmothers and shamans opened and reconnected me in so many ways; it was like a fast track. It was a few months after this that I would take my first sacred trip to Egypt and have my first full Akashic experience.

What Is the Akashic?

Think about a library in the universe. Think about a matrix of light that connects all energy—including you. The Akashic collects all the records and holds the book and story of your past life, present life, and future life.

Stand still for just a moment and think—how vast, how immense, and how amazing. Stand and stare up at the night sky, and you will see your gaze never ends. It truly is an infinite space around us and so, beloved, so are you!

The Akashic field acts as an energetic matrix, which is also known as the book of life. The word *Akashic* comes from *akasha* (the energy from which all life is formed).

When teaching, I refer to it as the ever-knowing space and place of time, but most importantly, as the library of life or book of records.

There are two ways of thinking about this, if you can understand the universe has a database and each of us is a file.

If each of us is a data file, we hold records in that file. The Akashic is the master file; all you need to know is the security code to connect or dial in. When teaching, I always ask who has a mobile phone, and virtually the whole room will place their hands in the air. I continue that if we understand that mobile phones connect through transmitters and we can dial a foreign country and talk to someone on the other side of the world, it is also possible that our brains and energy systems can act as transmitters.

Akasha, I believe, is the creation and the synthesis of our mental, physical, emotional, and spiritual responses to life.

Connecting to the frequency of akasha, you find your essence, and the therapy is created through accessing actions such as compassion, forgiveness, respect, release, and bringing of peace to all records that still hold trauma or distress.

That is the science part of the story; now here is the esoteric story as I saw in my first experience with this amazing new world of information and insight.

My first encounter of working in the Akashic field was on my first trip to Egypt. I remember I visited the pyramids at Giza as a tourist. When we reached the entrance, I refused to enter the Great Pyramid, as it felt inappropriate, and I could not explain at the time, but I felt it lacked ceremony of special preparation.

Instead my friend and I took a guided tour around Giza plateau. The Egyptian guide led us across the sand behind the pyramid and down toward the Sphinx, into an area where no other tourists seemed to be venturing. He led us down into a small walkway of tunnels under the pyramids, explaining that this was where the Americans were doing keyhole surgery to locate further tombs and temple sites. Sure enough, you could see where the small holes were located on the walls with chalk numbers and messages left.

He then did something strange: he placed me face-first against the wall. He stretched out my arms and hands and then gently pressed the palms of my hands into the cold, damp wall and placed my forehead and temple against the flat white stone. Then he took my friend for a tour of the caverns and left me standing, holding myself against this wall.

At first my head started to question. *This is crazy. It's freezing. I'm going to be covered in this stupid white dust. Crazy man and silly me.*

Then I relaxed. *Oh well,* I thought and laughed to myself, *another story to entertain with at the dinner table.* I began to smile and not take the incident so seriously, and at that point, my awareness shifted. I closed my eyes and could see a cavern in front of me—a long, dark tunnel. There, peering back at me, were two large, black, wolflike guardians holding spears with the ankh symbols at the top. They appeared like characters from a movie, and I was rooted to the spot in fear. But all they did was stare back and peer down at me.

I took a deep breath and tried to ground myself and pray like crazy that these were not demons sent to carry me off. When the guide returned, he peeled me off the wall and smiled. I was cold and covered in shiny white dust. When we reached the daylight, I shivered but sparkled from this covering of what appeared to be crystal dust.

I kept this story to myself until I visited Glastonbury for the first time and spent time with a woman who was to be my new teacher.

I stayed in a small retreat center, which was located on the sacred Tor site in Glastonbury. This is a place of extraordinary energy, where the Arthurian legends were created. Mary Magdalene is fabled to have lived there a short time, and for many it is known as the Heart Chakra of the planet.

Heart chakra it may be; however, Glastonbury is also a place of love, light, and shadow. Many who make a pilgrimage to heal their heart often have to deal with the reasons their heart is having difficulty opening. This can often happen in a very fast-track and uncomfortable way.

But this is the place I learned to truly be myself and open my heart, and this was the key to everything. Once I worked fully from this place, everything came thick and fast.

One day while I was visiting for a Flower of Life workshop, I asked my new teacher about my Egyptian experience. I shared with her the tale of the guardians, to which she nodded and appeared to understand. The white dust, she explained, had been my ancient initiation back into the ways of the priests and priestesses of the Giza plateau.

She did raise an eyebrow when I mentioned about my encounter with a funny-looking stone, which stood on a certain wall in the Cairo Museum.

"Ah, the consciousness stone," she said. "It found you?"

"Yes," I replied.

I told her about the Sunday afternoon when rambling through the Cairo Museum when I had been drawn toward a rather odd white square stone box on the wall. It felt like a magnet pulling me close, but it had no description and was listed nowhere on the tour guide. I felt it had connected with me and made me dizzy being so close to it.

My teacher explained this had come from Atlantis and had been left in Egypt to hold sacred records. It could also connect individuals with the cosmic energy. She suggested we should return and pay a visit. I agreed, and the following month, I traveled with thirty-two others on my first sacred journey through the Nile Valley. I admit I felt like a computer having a daily upgrade of my database and programs. These, I now realize, were my initiations and attunements.

Let me explain: we all carry healing energy within us, like tiny magnets or electricity running through our veins. When we clear our energy field and have an attunement to such things as Reiki, this switches the electricity on. The symbols, which are placed into you in the initiation, stay within you. Therefore, when you enter sacred sites or meditation, the guardians can read these invisible symbols and track the energy. It's very much like being given an access code chip or a cosmic passport.

Many people are born with abilities but never have their codes activated. Egypt activated many soul initiations during the ancient times; each temple had a specific purpose and teaching during a person's lifetime. Egyptians at that time knew that they were part of a reincarnation cycle, and each time they fulfilled an initiation, they would ascend to the next level of consciousness.

In part four of this book, I lead you through an Egyptian meditation, gently flowing through each sacred site, starting with the Root at Abu Simbel and then work to clear karma from each temple. As we travel, we re-activate the teaching that was created there and align it to your chakra line.

My first Akashic therapy work occurred during a group visit to the Egyptian Philae Temple, when I began to experience visions and flashbacks of past-life stories.

Philae is the temple of Isis and the divine feminine. It is so sacred to the Egyptian people that they endeavor to make a pilgrimage at least once in their lifetime.

During my first visit, I was present with the group for prayer and meditation. Then we all wandered to the location on the site that resonated with us. A small group of five women stood beside me near a small area of stairs. They began to have their own past-life recall. Some of them began to cry and looked in fear. Suddenly, my clairvoyant sight opened, and I began to work with them to heal and give forgiveness to whatever was bringing them grief. At first I thought these were my past lives, but I realized I could not be involved in all these times. So how on earth did I know what to say and do?

It would take three more sacred journeys to Egypt to lift the veils on my story, ability, and soul purpose of working with the Akashic. Once I realized this, I attracted more who were greatly helped by this teaching.

I continued further field research to other sacred sites, using the knowledge from various holistic therapies and metaphysical teachings to create a session. This appeared to fulfill the intention of healing, clearing, and gaining clarity from soul lives. So from this platform, Akashic therapy was created.

WHAT IS AKASHIC THERAPY?

Akashic Therapy examines the past, present, life between lives, and future lives for healing, clearing, and clarity. It is often defined as a metaphysical concept as it relates to the transcendent or to a reality beyond what is perceptible to the senses. It is mainly observed by the etheric or clair senses.

> **Clairvoyant** – *visual. To see information, I sometimes allow my vision to wander and become blurred. In meditation, the pictures show me the messages.*
>
> **Clairsentient** – *feeling. Describing how you feel in session or meditation is valuable. A sense of fear or joy indicates the karmic level in the session. Where the body feels emotion is also relevant, as certain parts of the body or chakra regions give an indication of areas to clear.*
>
> **Clairaudient** – *hearing. The messages, often words appear in the client's mind, or whispers that mention names or places guide a session.*
>
> **Claircognizant** – *knowing. This is the trusting sense of resonance. In session, there are sometimes moments when everything feels, sounds, and looks right, as if it was meant to be.*

The Akashic session was created by me to engage with clients to assist them in reading their Akashic records. These clair- senses help to heal, clear, and give clarity to all aspects of the information stored in the books of your soul journey.

THE AKASHIC THERAPY METHOD

The regression and progression under hypnosis is used in many forms of psychotherapy by professionals to uncover subconscious thought and change beliefs, which are challenging to the lifestyle of the individual.

Akashic therapy begins with an ancient Divine Heart meditation. This meditation from the sacred feminine initiation allows the client to open their heart and answer questions from the subconscious without fear or ego. This depth of connection often touches on the real place of superconsciousness within us.

Akashic therapy does not use names or specific dates; therefore, the confusion of famous archetypes does not occur. Ego is not necessary for this work. We work to heal the records, not to simply view and relive.

I try to avoid a clinical method and create an environment which allows the client to relax and drift into an amazing vision.

I sometimes try to find music that resonates with Egypt and the Akashic library. In a personal conversation with past life regression expert Brian Weiss, he informed me that of all the places most people connect a past life record is to a life in ancient Egypt or Atlantis.

During the Akashic session, I create an etheric pod connection to the King's Chamber in the Great Pyramid on Giza plateau. When I visited this space with groups on the equinoxes, after the private ceremony, my role was to escort the initiates into the chariot or stone chamber within the room. Once this chariot has been energetically opened with Reiki symbols and key ancient Egyptian words, the energy activates, and initiates can connect back to their soul star or the energy of the universe for a few short minutes. This works like an elevator as I connect the grounding cords, open the sky veil, and wrap the client in etheric ribbons to keep them connected and safe. When they return, they feel a sense of belonging and connection to the earth; they liken it to a womblike experience.

You can be in sacred sites, nature, and your own home, and results can still be obtained. You will feel safe and a clear connection to yourself and the universe. These sessions are rich in life lessons and mind-body-spirit experience. As one of my friends experienced:

CASE STUDY DIANE

I lay within the Chariot and closed my eyes. Immediately I left my body and was propelled into deep space. Infinite blackness, surrounded by golden stars and symbols. Absolute peace and beauty. Then, sound, the most beautiful angelic tones coming, it seemed, from beyond space and time. Then a flicker of memory and I knew I had to return or would never find my way back. I opened my eyes and leaning over the top of the chariot were various faces, calling me back. Slowly I returned, managed to stand and climb out barely able to stand, totally moved by the beauty of the experience. The next person took their place and I joined the other women to tone over the sarcophagus. This was a beautiful experience as it felt familiar, memories of past lives as priestesses flooded in. So gentle, subtle and absolutely female. I am so very grateful and continue to be moved by the experience. I will never forget it.

Thank you Amanda, what you shared and the beautiful way that you work moves me still.

WHY AKASHIC THERAPY?

Taking an Akashic journey works with the four key areas of conscious and subconscious life. It is these areas which we strive to keep in balance. This way we attract positive opportunities, peace, and happiness into our lives. We often start by repairing our physical bodies and stretching our educated minds; however, we sometimes loose focus on the emotional and spiritual aspects. This is where deep issues settle and ferment, causing sadness, illness, and pain. This sickening lies low and hidden throughout lifetimes until the individual is ready for it to heal.

Akashic therapy works with all these aspects of the soul journey. It shines a light to bring healing, clearing, and clarity. Let me explain how with the aspects of spiritual, emotional, mental, and physical.

Spiritual

The Akashic journey enables you to connect with your guides and access the information to help you on your spiritual path. Having this earth experience can be confusing; so many things do not make rational sense. However, in spiritual practice, all is calm and makes perfect sense. The Akashic will allow you to retrieve the tools and messages that support this journey and quickly help heal the issues that can be holding you back. It also can do this without going round and round the story or he said/she said, going to the core issue and bringing back a peaceful solution. It is then, however, the choice of the individual whether they follow their heart. This heart space allows the intuition part of us to grow.

I am often asked when do people find their spirituality, and I normally reply, "When they are five minutes from dying and passing over."

For this is a time when nothing else and no one else matters. You are entering another phase of life, but in an energy form. It is at this point the subconscious takes over and the mind gives up and just accepts.

In this time of change and awakening, many are following their hearts and looking at life through a different lens. This was all written in many sacred texts, and many have seen it with their visions. Being on my spiritual path changed my beliefs and thought patterns; it takes me from fear to love and helps me make conscious choices, which serve many, not just myself.

Akashic therapy can unlock and awaken your spiritual gifts achieved from a past life that lies dormant and silent. On one occasion in Dendara Temple in Egypt, I worked with a group of women in the crypt area below the temple. It is a small, dark cavern with hidden messages of love, life, and passion. One woman recalled her experience for me and what this Akashic initiation had unlocked for her.

While in the crypt with you and during the initiation I didn't have any visions or remembrances, it all happened a bit later. At Karnak one of the temple guardians pulled me to one side after we had all been to see Sekmeth and asked me to wait till everyone had left. He then motioned me to go and spend 2-3 minutes alone with Sekmeth. A while later I found myself roaring out loud like a lioness! He touched the base of my spine. I felt then that it had to do with my Kundalini energy. Now Krishna has appeared in my life and is teaching me new forms of Kundalini meditation. So every morning I start with a meditation to raise the Kundalini energy. Isn't that amazing. Happened all after your initiation in Dendara! THANK YOU!

Emotional

Past-life Karma and the Karma of loved ones can create toxins and shock, which return in future lives. It waits until a similar situation returns to play, either with another soul or another episode on your journey. Then the emotional toxin comes into play; it often shows itself in the form of grief or distress and comes at you like a wave. The Akashic therapy brings these to the surface in story form, to allow you to witness the journey without reliving it. This enables change and healing. This is an amazing healing tool with victims of abuse and allows the individual to move on from being the victim.

The key words of the emotion surface in the session. Sometimes the client will feel them, but not to the extent that it takes over the session.

We release the negative emotions and replace them with positive responses. Forgiveness and compassion are the key emotional responses worked with in this area—forgiveness and compassion for the client and situation from which they are emotionally distressed.

I've witnessed people behave with anger, rage, fear, passion, and deep love upon meeting new people in sacred sites. They have little recollection afterward, except that it stirs a deep emotion within them. When we examine their time before in this site or with this person, we find they have indeed suppressed great emotion and have not healed or cleared the Karma. I have encountered those who, in anger, have created curses, which they later have to undo and ask forgiveness for. If not cleared, these curses can show themselves in future lifetimes.

Mental

Often our limiting beliefs and mental blocks can feed our fear and ego. As we know, the mind can play tricks and often brings its friends, sabotage and self-pity, to the party.

Akashic therapy is assisted by the mental state in forming images or recalling words and affirmations in order to rewire the records with healing and peace and not negativity. It is my belief that we cannot change the records, but we can interpret them in a greater, more positive way. In sessions, we have never changed events, merely changed the reaction and comprehension.

Your divine heart does not feed these little negative energies, but your mind sometimes does. Once you have warmed that heart and connected, you know you are part of a greater picture. You have life and purpose and divine worth. Then the mind calms and creates the details and stories and helps you understand these in a loving and learning format.

Physical

The Akashic can show why we have manifested certain physical diseases and aliments. These conditions in others or in ourselves are created to trigger calls to action. Once we know why this disease is holding on to our physical selves, we can work toward healing and clearing it faster and safer.

We can incarnate carrying the injuries of the past; clients will often comment of neck or back pain. When we have journeyed back into the Akashic, we find a sword or axe has been the issue, and they still carry the cellular knowledge that recreates an effect in this life. A session can help gently remove this and heal the etheric energy, to allow the physical body to get to work. When you live in truth, your body flourishes.

When the subconscious is ignored or silenced, the body no longer has a voice and can choose to regress.

I always find Louise Hay's "heal your body" crib sheet book is essential for this work. Placing positive intentions and affirmation with the Akashic assists the recovery process.

When all these aspects of ourselves are in balance, it is amazing the progress we make and what we attract toward us. I have also found the Akashic an amazing place to find and draw inspiration. For a while, a great deal of my clients were writers, some new and some established and famous on the New York Times bestseller list. When I took them on an Akashic journey, they often returned with new ideas or concepts for plot or character. I was once with a new writer who asked many questions about my work and the Akashic and how to find her passion. We commented about her fears of writing and topics and styles of writing. It was at this point I suddenly stopped and asked her to go into her heart. This lady had worked a great deal on her soul purpose work and was therefore very connected and in my opinion ready to channel many other spiritual dimensions. I opened up the garden sanctuary and asked her about writing from a past life. "Byron" was the name she came back with. I brought her back out of the session, as this appeared to be the message. We spent a few moments thinking about Byron's work and how that energy stream could help her work. The Akashic can make introductions to amazing mentors and teachers for divine connections that can be creative and inspiring.

I am often asked what is true etheric communication and another person's ego talking. In my experience, when the true etheric channel starts, you feel a change in the energy around you, and their voice or face alters. The information is always of a high-vibration language; they always bring the message back to love and peace.

One such lady had an amazing, uplifting session and shared with me her thoughts and emotions.

CASE STUDY ANGELA

Our session on Sunday I have to say has lingered in my consciousness and left me quite speechless on how amazing it was, and its effect on me, so I think it's helpful for me to have the chance to write a few things about it, integrating the experience a bit further.

Not knowing much about working with the Akashic records, I wasn't sure how it would all pan out and was amazed to see how much I ended up getting from it.

I absolutely loved everything about the session; the visualization you facilitated was great in preparing to enter the two doors, one to the matrix and the second to the Akashic records. I loved the significance of the butterflies and the colored flowers that played later on in the session and at the very end when these two symbols came back again to play their part into my journey. As I didn't know anything about the matrix and the golden highway, it was great to see you were recognizing the places I was entering, contextualizing my experience, and giving it meaning and grounding it for me.

In fact you seemed to know and recognize every part of the journey I was going through, not only visually, but metaphysically, mentally, spiritually, emotionally, even when at times I was having complex experiences. You seemed to be aware of my experiences as I was having them, recognizing and often able to intuit what I was feeling but was not able to put into words. That made me feel held and supported but also showed me this is a trodden path not unique to me but to many, reminding me the universality of our human experience. Yes we're all having our unique experiences, yet they happen within the same matrix of beingness. All walking the golden highway. I find this very moving.

On another hand, the scientist in me found this journey exciting as an exercise to metaphysical anatomy of the universal structures that I used to read about yet not experiencing myself. So that was also very interesting to me. Yet as the experience was complex I was unable to find words. In fact you just seemed to be able to pin it completely and with great accuracy, helping me make meaning of my experience.

You were sensitive to your guidance, in a way that though you guided, it was still I paving the path and making sense of things, giving me a helping hand when I needed it in an appropriate way. I was also surprised to see the energy vibration had heightened significantly during the session, feeling you had tapped into a really big energy source that made everything more conscious and the experience more easily understood.

EXERCISES

Sit down with a pen and paper
and write at the top:

*I am safe, I am connected to the universal
source, I have all the information within me.*

Now write down these categories:
Past Life
Life Between Life
Present Life
Future Life

Now place one question under each of these headings, asking what you desire to know or are curious about. The purpose of these exercises is to open up your channels of communication and loosen you up.

They also place a start of intention and focus toward the information being delivered later on in the book, when you encounter the meditations.

Now also ask yourself the questions:

Why does Akashic work attract and resonate with you?

What would you like to know about these areas of your soul database?

Write your answers, thoughts, or even further questions.

Do not worry about your answers; some may surprise you, enlighten you, or confuse you. Just trust yourself, dear one, and begin to open the doorway to your heart.

Where Does the Akashic Journey Go?

Imagine we are standing on the planet Earth and can touch the grass, feel the wind, and see the sun. This is known as the third dimension. It's our first level of consciousness and our first reference point.

After this, the veils of dimensions turn thinner and finer in the energy level. The fourth dimension, I would say, is where things around us move, but the visual is weaker and requires clairvoyant sight to see. These dimensions then go up in number, higher in vibration and purity. The angels, I believe live between the fourth and fifth dimensions.

As we become more aware of these dimensions and work in the Akashic zones, we too take on some of the characteristics of these other dimensions. We become sensitive to toxins and frequencies that do not nurture or serve us.

The Akashic is a realm between the worlds. It is the record-storage area, and we access it through the energy or electric grids that flow like a matrix around the universe.

Imagine the globe in your mind and see it wrapped in a golden grid and every cross of the grid is a point you can visit with your subconscious.

While working with a university professor who was working on a PhD, I explored this golden matrix. His topic of study was heritage and ancient sites for tourism. He could not explain in full about this certain location he was about to visit and feature. I suggested we visit through the Akashic method and connect to the energy grid.

First we took him to a sacred place in his heart, through

the sanctuary garden and then to this ancient location. On a large piece of paper I recorded his journey for him.

At first he felt very comfortable and navigated the area, describing to me where the doorways and stairs led. He spent some time watching the activity on this site. He could recall the smell and feel of the place. He was able to talk about this site as a living area full of people and purpose. This was no longer a tourist site but a place where he felt he had lived a past life. He had promised to protect and care for this beautiful part of the world. The area was in North Africa, and he became very excited when talking about the bazaars and traders. Although his eyes were closed, his face was animated and alive.

We looked at how this place affected all his senses, why he was connected with this location, what may happen to this place in the future, and the contribution his PhD work would provide. After the session, we had so many words, phrases, and points of reference. He also had a deeper understanding and knowledge of this site, which developed the writing and enhanced the visiting experience.

Sometimes clients will visit to look at their internal energy bodies, their Chakra system, and aura.

As in all things, you can go outward or inward. Some clients who have had illness feel comfortable enough to visit the internal body organs and systems. In session, the client will describe the color or the feeling they have around this part of the body. We send love and place a positive affirmation into this area. I find that this helps clients when they then visit their medical doctors, because they are taking medical advice and support but also feel they have knowledge and personal empowerment with their physical body.

This is something greater
Created around me
Drawing positive energy and light
This radiates through me
Connecting me to my highest good
I choose to release my past
Now I heal all my karma
I observe my story
I am creating wisdom in my heart
I am setting myself free to love

PART TWO

Using the Akashic Therapy

When to Begin?

Your journey can start today, right here, right now. All you have to do is make a sacred contract with yourself—a contract that for a few moments or more, you will open your heart to the magnificent universe and allow yourself to heal, clear, and gain clarity for your life in this lifetime.

This is the affirmation I have on my wall when I am working with the Akashic:

I allow my heart energy and soul to heal, clear, and gain clarity through the lifetimes past, present, and future. I am connected to the universe in a beautiful, blissful, and balanced way. Each day brings joy and happiness, knowledge, wisdom, and peace around me.

You can work on your own affirmation; think about the intention and why you would want to read your records. You can achieve this work alone or with an Akashic buddy. You read the meditations for them and they read the meditations for you.

COMMON BLOCKS

Your limiting beliefs and fear can be the key things that block your journey. It takes an open mind and an open heart to reach into the unknown and take the leap of faith into the truth.

We all choose to place our heads in the sand at some times on our spiritual paths, but those who look up and reach to the stars have the best sunrise and sunset views in their lives.

Working from the mind can block your access to the Akashic records. I remember working with an amazing hypnotherapist and observing her work with a client. She took her client back through the steps and counts, keeping the mind focused on the hypnotic procedure. All of a sudden, the girl's energy changed, and her body started to shake. She was going into fear.

My colleague tried to reassure her as she started to cry and say fearfully, "It's dark and things are moving. I think I've gone to a bad place."

We waited a little longer as I saw a different storyline running and just raised my hand gently to ask if I could take over. This girl was lying on the bed, unable to speak or move forward. I knew that if we woke her at this stage, she may remain in this recurring flashback nightmare. I felt confident in my vision for her. I knew she was really in a safe place. My colleague gently started to mention my name, and I carefully stepped into the guiding role.

"Lydia, can you hear me?" I whispered. "I'm here to guide you back through," I reassured her.

"I'm scared, it's dark, and I think I'm in a bad place," she cried.

"Okay, well, you do not belong there," I reassured her. "But before we come back, just stop a moment and breathe. Know you are safe, and look down at your feet."

"They are on dark, spongy grass," she said.

"Okay, and what else is around?" I inquired.

"Trees, stumps, and branches," she answered, amused.

"Where are you, Lydia? Just breathe and stay in your heart. Relax," I said.

By this time, I had aligned all my angels around her and asked for support.

"Oh, I see little flowers and things floating," she said. She was still lying flat, her eyelids the only thing moving. "Oh, it's fairies and elves, and they live here," she said, excited.

My colleague and I breathed relief and smiled. I went on to take her on a magical journey into the elemental kingdom from which we found her energy resonated.

When she came out of session and we grounded her energy back home, she admitted she thought she had gone to the lower astral plane, or hell, as many would describe it. She knew she had gone to a home place, and the idea that it was this dark space terrified her. We learnt a great deal that day. Trusting intuition and stepping out of fear can save the day.

Every day we are listening for the messages around us, as humans, we are often afraid of the silence and meditation process. However, these are moments when we truly connect with the divine in us and around us. Our intuition finds a voice, and our flow of life expands.

On the amazing island of Roatan off the coast of Honduras, I have found the ocean and crystal energy amazing for helping clients focus and develop awareness. One gifted lady, Maria, had spent time on this island and placed her trust in Akashic therapy.

CASE STUDY MARIA

The Akashic reading you guided me with was most helpful at the time. It was my first experience with Akashic methods.

Having a hard time then with meditating I felt with your guidance this was quite a unique approach. The experience helped me understand better that my personal guides are very present with a unique message each. The channeling was clear and showed me how the universe is connected.

Today I am learning to meditate and at times reach a level where I can reach my own subconscious path. Your session made me more aware how connected we are to present and past. It brought me closer on how to reach my own soul's purpose. If I am quiet I reach that point at times. During the day and night I see and read the messages that come out of seemingly nowhere. I do not look for them. They appear at the right time and moment for me to understand. Not always to act on. Just being in the moment.

My reasons for being and experiencing where I was in this life became more in view. In general I started to see the total picture. For me it was a process of letting go on all levels. I was aware that blocks had to be removed first. Both you and other methods helped me with removal and restructuring.

Once I let go and did not think of what's next the most amazing things started to happen and are still happening. Trusting and knowing I am guided in this process once so hard now so easy. Having met my guides during that session makes me reach back to them as if they are on this planet. This I do when I catch myself holding on.

> *Things have shifted for me. Several people who had not seen me for a long time asked me if I had lost weight. No I feel lighter. But nice to be noticed. I'm so blessed to live in this world today.*

Once we allow our intuition to open within us, the blocks to the other dimensions fall away. We begin to use all our senses and move toward relationships and situations that bring joy and happiness.

The universe is limitless in its creativity, and so are we.

EXERCISE

Take a piece of paper and allow yourself to open the door to your ego. For a few minutes, write down the fear, reservations, and concerns you have. You can use Oracle or Angel cards for clarity.

When you have listed this, take a moment and ask your heart if this is truth or illusion. For many facing these fears, it is a leap of faith. Now take a deep breath and begin to say the affirmation:

I welcome every experience as part of my evolution.
I am now clearing my negative beliefs.
I am dissolving barriers.
I am safe in the flow of life.

Use this affirmation over and over again, and revisit the blocks and see how they make no sense. When you are ready to release them, scratch them out. Draw a heart around them and release them.

TRUST AND INTUITION

I always start a session with a positive intention. Trust is also a vital tool for gaining clarity.

I trust myself and hold truth in my heart.

Trust, I feel, is often like a sacred flame that wraps around us, runs through us, and from which we walk through our greatest fears to embrace a greater love for ourselves. It offers a state of being in grace and peace. Our minds can often clutter this with sabotage and victim role-play.

Our gut feeling is the survival instinct and a skill we have lost or closed over our years of growing up and integrating into our social norms.

Trust in others is a mirror. When I can't trust others, I'm really saying I can't trust myself. Others can surprise us in unusual, amazing, or heartbreaking ways. This is the ground of great learning and testing. How do we hold that moment when a loved one deceives us or we feel abandoned by them? These are natural reactions as we stumble through the forest of life. In shaman traditions, they teach that for every poison, thirteen steps away is the cure. Know and trust that the rebalance is there. Many of us follow lifetimes of never trusting a cure for happiness.

But how does one reach this state of trust utopia? The answer is clear: it's a mixture of heart and truth. When our hearts are open, our minds still, and we speak or just know our truth, the trust comes—trust in others, the universe, and ourselves.

And in the end, a deeper knowing and greater grace develop, you become one with your world, and the sacred flame of trust supports you, guides you, and shines brighter than the sun to attract an abundance of trust to you, with you, and from you.

Take some time to connect with your heart. This is the vital part of working within the Akashic realm. It will help your intuition and allow you to trust the messages and guidance you receive.

You can open your own clairvoyant transmitter to the universe and others around you and develop your intuitive skills.

EXERCISES

Close your eyes for a moment and think about the last hour of your day. When ready, open your eyes and write down a description of what you remember.

Write what you *saw, heard, felt, and understood;* what was going on around you. As you recall the information, you will notice which is your first, second, third, and fourth sense.

- Which sense created the most information?
- Which information do you trust and resonate with?

This is an exercise to help you explore your senses which are dominant and give you confidence in the Akashic meditations. The "previous hour" episode you know to be true. You trust the information. As you practice working with your Akashic records, you too will develop this deeper intuition of knowing and truth.

CREATING SACRED SPACE

Creating sacred space is very important; your whole vibration and energy need to be at peace and ready for your journey.

Sacred space means safety and allows you to take responsibility for your journey. When you fill the space in which you work with divine light and love, a great bubble of protection surrounds you. This bubble acts as a filter to allow high energy to reach you. It deflects anything negative or non-serving away from you.

It is always important to create your own sacred space when having an Akashic session by yourself or with others. It does not have to be a whole room dedicated for the occasion, but there are key elements that can clear and heal the energy and vibration around you. It can also protect the session and lift you to a higher vibration to obtain messages and connections with these levels.

Here are a few of the key elements that I use.

Candles and flame burn any negative energy and keep the light around you.

Lighting should be soft and gentle. When the light is dimmed, it allows the third eye to focus and look past the 3D frame into the clairvoyant space.

Music from a sound healer is fantastic to take your brainwave state into a calm dream trance. (Remember not to use this while driving or at work.) There are some great sites from which you can download various wave sounds that resonate with you.

Water to drink or a water feature allows a level of flow and purity. I find working near the ocean a great way to let the images flow and go. The ocean waves bring the information gently forward, and then, as you release, it takes it straight to the ocean bed and Gaia, who transmutes the negative forces. Pictures of water also work; waterfall images are perfect.

The **four directions** are often used in indigenous tribal and ancient ceremony. You can place crystals in the corners of the room or ask an angel to hold space. Often before starting, you can acknowledge the guides from the four corners of the Earth to support you and guide you.

Singing bowls and bells hold a tone and sound pitch, which clears the energy around us and can signal the start or end of a session. It's important to open with respect for the Akashic stream and close with honor. The high pitch of sound can break the cord gently, to help you ground back into your safe space.

Warmth and comfort are essential at all times. We are spiritual beings having an earthbound experience. On sacred journeys, I am always vigilant of others who are "out of body." While this is safe in a group, often when we return to daily life, it can leave us bewildered and scared to venture out from the cocoon. Always create a safe space or an affirmation to reground you and bring you back into a present space, place and time.

Creating a sacred space on the outside often asks that we create on the inside. What we create internally often mirrors and attracts our environment.

Remember to honor your body and energy on a regular basis. Akashic work heals on such a deep level, your physical body may need recharging after a session.

Water and herbal tea can cleanse daily toxins, as can massage and sea-salt baths. Walking outside is wonderful to clear your head and the cobwebs of the mind. This will help you to connect and flow with the energy. I have also found that after the Akashic work, grounding food supports your physical body. When in Egypt after temple or session work I find tea, potato dishes, bread, nuts, and soups also help. Hot chocolate or cacao drinks are excellent for calming the soul and nourishing the spirit. Doing Akashic work may not burn calories, but it certainly uses up energy, and a little sugar or fruit can help you through. Listen to your body and check out what it feels it needs.

Many sessions often take you to historic and sacred sites. This can be a confusing area, as you may be connecting with these energy streams or it may have been you or your past life.

Historic Characters

Sometimes I have people who come for the Akashic video show, just to see if they can see something from another lifetime. Working with the Akashic is not about feeding your ego, and if you're looking to see yourself as a historic, famous, or infamous character, this is not the right space. Famous people will often present themselves during a session, but I have encountered a great many Cleopatras and Napoleons to know that not all can be that person. This is your subconscious way of communicating the type of life character or archetype that needs releasing, clearing, or healing. If these people appear in meditations, look at the lesson or message they bring to you.

Sacred Sites

When we walk through a temple, there are three ways you can read energy in a sacred space. These sacred spaces are imprinted with high levels of energy that you can connect with in various ways.

- You could be the person who walked in this temple and remembered a past life.
- You are picking up the energy that was imprinted before.

- The spirit of the ancient one is still walking with you.

It is important to see the lesson and teaching and not become lost in the story. Akashic work is about moving the past over and clearing through the present to reach a peaceful, joyous future.

When connecting or walking in these amazing areas, one needs to be observant of the imprint one is leaving. Be an observer and hold an intention to only leave footprints of peace and happiness behind you.

Open Your Heart with Meditation

One of the essential parts of Akashic work is about being in your heart. The Heart Energy or Heart Chakra acts as a window to your soul and a filter of your inner knowing. Your heart holds your deep secrets and brilliance.

When clients visit for their first Akashic work, we spend time bringing this sacred heart to life. We connect it to the universal source. When this first happens, it is an amazing experience, and tears often flow as if a great release has occurred.

This meditation should be performed as regularly as possible. After a while, your whole consciousness resonates with the process. Then it's a simple smile, relax, and on hearing the words "Go into your heart," you transcend into a place of balance, bliss, and beauty.

This is the key to unlocking the door to all your inner knowing. You may wish to keep a journal that records the experiences of working with your heart.

Divine Heart Meditation

This is required before any Akashic session. Your eyes can be open or closed. Sometimes I record the meditation to replay then I can close my eyes.

Now we begin.
Find a comfortable space to sit and relax.
Gently take three deep breaths from the solar
plexus (lower stomach) breathe them out.
Relax and allow your attention to wander to your heart.

Imagine a bright light growing in your heart
and spreading throughout your body.
See the light move down your lower body and
down through your legs, through your feet, and
like tree roots all the way into the earth.
See your roots of shining light reach
the crystal of Gaia and connect.
As you do, you see the crystal sparkle and the
light rise back up though the roots into your
feet, legs, and body, back to the heart.
See the light rise from your heart and move
through your throat into your head, and like a
fountain, allow it to move up through your head
into the sky and connect with a star above.
See the light move back to you until the pulse
remains in your heart and the light that surrounds
you is a column from sky to earth.
Now focus on your heart and let's warm it awake.
Imagine it has a glowing star with five points.
To open all the points, allow the heart energy to flow and
focus on the happiest moments or people in your life.
Relax and smile, and let the happy
thoughts expand this heart chakra.
Send light around this star.
Feel your shoulders relax back, and
feel the peace around you.
Now see a small flame in the center of the star.
Allow yourself to flow into the flame.
This is the flame of transformation and transmutation;
it clears negativity and brings purification and clarity.

Warm yourself in the flame and smile.
Now look down and see a pearl, a beautiful
translucent and radiant pearl.
Hold it in your hand, gently send it love,
and be amazed at how beautiful it is.
This is your heart, beloved, your divine heart.
The perfect essence of yourself when
you were created as a star seed.
And this is now the place you can visit and ask your truth.
You are connected to the earth and
universe and in your divine heart.
So now, beloved, what is it you wish to know?

Allow yourself just to relax in the moment and close your eyes again for five minutes.
See what gently comes to you.

Record your experiences in your special notebook.

- How did you feel?
- What did you connect with?
- How does your heart feel?

Who Are My Guides?

If you read any esoteric guides to the dimensions and etheric planes, you will find that there are many different levels around the universe that hold unique types of energies. It is these energies or guides, as we call them, who can step forward to support you. They connect with you when you enter this sacred part of yourself. In my experience, I often sense an energy approaching before the client but have learned to stay back as an observer and facilitator. I allow the contact to be created. Over the years, this has taken many different forms. Here are a few of the most prominent guides who have stepped forward so kindly to help with Akashic therapy and how to connect with them.

Angels

With each of us is a guardian angel. They are assigned when our soul reincarnates into this earth realm. They walk beside us every step of the way. They are unable to step forward unless requested and are on strict contract not to interfere with our earthly choices.

Your angels understand and know what lies in front, behind, and all around you. They can often make themselves known to you by leaving signatures such as white feathers. Sometimes the word *angel* appears in a book, magazine article or even a song on the radio. I find the best way to have a conversation with them is with Oracle cards. Angel Oracle cards work by providing a personal life coach and direct telephone line. You can ask a question, and amazing angels such as Michael or Gabriel will step forward. This often gives a great indication as to where your Akashic session will be guided. The angel message cards can give the information as to the type of lesson or contract that needs to be healed. I'm often an impatient channel, but in my experience, the angelic realm likes this direct response and relates with greater clarity to enable the session to progress.

An affirmation to connect with the angels:

Angel light is all around me; I am safe, supported and Love. My angel wings are ready to fly.

Spirit Guides

Many of us have native guides or gurus with whom we have walked in our previous earth lives. Quite often, I will find I'm working with a certain guide who is familiar to the client. I will describe this guide as I see them, and the client joins in the conversation also. Spirit guides act as teachers of knowledge and wisdom. They appear when a person is ready for new direction and needs information regarding the genre of teaching they require.

An affirmation to connect with spirit guides:

My spirit guides show me wisdom and knowledge to guide my journey with joy and happiness; I welcome them into my life.

Friends and Family—Loved Ones

Loved ones who have passed over often find they return to their roles of angels or guides for those still on the earth plane.

Often when a client is working in their first session, a parent or grandparent who has passed will step forward. This can be emotional but also very comforting. This often happens when we work in the "present-life" realm, as family and loved ones can leave without a final good-bye. This type of Akashic session is amazing to support the grieving process for you. It allows you to place a gentle good-bye or "see you later" into your records. Using the garden sanctuary of the Akashic, we are able to allow these guides to step forward. They can reassure us we are all safe and how they would like to help us. You are never alone again.

An affirmation to connect with family and loved ones:

I am connected to my family, I am loved through the generations, I welcome their love and support around me.

Ascended Masters

There are beings around us of highly evolved consciousness, which we refer to as masters. Kwan Yin, Buddha, and Jesus are often recalled in sessions of future lives. They show the soul learning for the future life. They also appear in the Akashic ashrams, which are like the schools of teaching we can go to in our life between life.

In 2008, I found everywhere I looked images of Mother Mary, everywhere blue, and a great many clients working with lives related around the stories of Jesus. On the March 2008 Egypt trip, when the journey had almost ended, I felt a strong urge to visit the Coptic area in Cairo. This journey had been totally focused on ancient Egypt up till this point. I did not want to confuse the group by bringing another journey into play. But I knew a connection needed to be made in this energetic place.

In my previous research, I knew Mary had connection with this area but I had no idea what, where, or why. I mentioned to a few other women that I was going and had booked a taxicab early the next day. I would visit the area and then be back before lunch and the daily group session. The next morning, three women were waiting in the reception area.

We ran to the taxis, an old black-and-white cab damaged on every side, but it had four wheels, an engine, and a driver who smiled from his heart. We made our way into the old area of Cairo just as it was waking. Chickens and life were running everywhere. It felt like we had stepped back in time. We allowed ourselves to be led around each of the churches; so many different faiths all in one small area. We walked silently into the mosques, synagogues, and Christian churches.

Our veils were on and off, and so many rosaries and cards were bought. Then suddenly we stopped and looked over at a small church.

"Can we wait a little?" said one of the group, and we stopped.

Adopting our tourist stance, we gently leaned against the wall.

"I can feel Mary," whispered one woman.

Indeed, a soft, gentle breeze floated by, and each one of us felt we had received a great and gentle healing. We all felt that she walked with each of us and would be with us when we needed guidance. We said prayers and blessed the churches and this place for its unity of light. Then we raced back to the group in the hotel in Giza. Upon returning, I immediately opened my computer. What was the connection? And why so strong?

Brilliant Google showed me the church we had been drawn to. It was the one in which Mary, Joseph, and Jesus had sought sanctuary when they left Bethlehem, when Herod was on his karmic mission.

And the day? Well, we had paid no attention. It was Good Friday.

These amazing masters of light are great teachers and

messengers of healing. You only have to invite and invoke their gifts into your life.

An affirmation to connect with ascended masters:

I have the infinite power of the universe within me. My higher self is guiding me toward the greater good. I resonate with divine and great beings. I welcome the wisdom into my whole beingness.

Light Beings from Other Planets

As our consciousness levels expand, so does our knowledge and awareness of other realms of life. Clients often report going home and bringing back messages from other solar systems. This sometimes causes distress for clients, as they still feel they are star people (souls still connected to other planets) or walk-ins (when a star soul has overtaken an earth-soul body with permission). Akashic therapy allows a window where you can explore this area without judgment. There is often a resonance between our souls and certain planets or star systems. They will make themselves known to you during sessions with words, symbols, or colors.

An affirmation to connect with light beings, planets, and star systems:

I am part of the cosmic golden matrix, I am energy of the light, I connect with ease and grace. I resonate with the universe around me.

Power Animals

Animals, sea life, and mythical creatures often appear with messages and guidance within Akashic sessions. Each animal is known as a totem. The Native Americans were amazing in their wisdom and information regarding why an animal had chosen to come to you and work with you. They taught what medicine or wisdom these creatures wished to share. Some power animals will appear for a certain healing or clearing, and some will walk with you always. Dolphins and whales are amazing energies to work with. Sometimes even Disney characters will appear to show you a message in picture animation form to help you understand.

An affirmation to connect with power animals:

I am one with nature; I honor all the creatures of the dimensions. I understand the messages they communicate.

Colors

During a session, I will often ask a client what color the flowers are and what color are they wearing. In meditation, the flowers you see indicate the chakra point that is holding the issue to resolve. The color of the butterflies indicates the chakra which is transforming with the Akashic therapy. If unsure where a shade of color is located, check on a color wheel chart. I often find pink falls into red, turquoise into blue.

Colors are used in the past, present, and future lives. I have not found that color occurs in the life between lives. This often appears a neutral area of blacks, whites, and grays with subtle shades.

This is a quick reference guide to the color and chakra points.

Color	Chakra	Meaning
Red	Root your base and perineum	Sexuality, security, possessions, obsessions, protection, connection to the earth.
Orange	Sacral, reproductive areas	Relationships, addictions, interaction, feminine energy.
Yellow	Solar plexus and stomach	Power, fear, self-knowledge and purpose, masculine energy, intellect.
Green	Heart and chest area	Passion, tenderness, inner-child energy, peace, harmony.
Blue	Throat and voice	Self-expression, will, communication, dreams, calming, creativity.
Indigo	Third eye and senses	Balance of lower- and higher-energy vibrations, clairvoyance, intuition, inspiration. Clarity.
Violet	Crown and knowing	Unity, claircognizance, transcending energy, wisdom, connection to the universe. Spiritual growth.
White	The area above your head which engages with your soul star	This is the soul star and the filter where all the spiritual knowledge keys and codes sit until you are ready to download, if you send gratitude, affirmations, and energy to this space above your head and see a shower of pure light rain down around you.

The Sanctuary Meditation

We will now work with the Sanctuary meditation to meet some of your guides.

Now sit down with pen and paper or your journal and write down the following categories.

- Angels
- Spirit Guides
- Friends and Loved Ones
- Ascended Masters
- Light Beings
- Power Animals

Select one group at a time to work with or leave the door open to opportunity.

Just relax.

Once you feel comfortable and your heart is open, you will feel radiance around you.

From here, we will work with the
Sanctuary meditation that follows.
Relax and breathe gently, and allow your
awareness to connect with your heart.

Allow the light from your heart to connect
to the center of the earth.
Allow this light to return back up
through your Chakra column.
Imagine yourself in a beautiful sanctuary garden.
See the green grass,
The blue sky.
The sun is shining.
See the flowers around you.
Watch the butterflies floating around you.

Imagine you are seated in the corner of the garden.
Across the garden, a wonderful, radiant light approaches.
Allow this light to take a form that resonates with you.
Feel the kindness and support around you.
Spend time with this beloved energy.
When ready, gently return to your present space.

Record your experience in your special notebook.

- How did you feel?
- What colors did you see? (This indicates the Chakra area from which you were working.)
- Who did you meet?
- What messages did they bring for you?
- Did they bring any gifts?
- How does your heart feel?

Now gently allow this meeting to pass, and become fully aware of your present space. It is important that you stay connected and grounded. Remember, you are here to have an earthly experience. Do not worry if you do not have a full visualization or someone unexpected shows up. You may find they appear in dreams or messages later in the day.

ENERGY LINES AND SACRED CONTRACTS

If we stop for a moment and imagine all the energy floating around us and imagine ourselves connected to that flow, we become linked to everyone and everything. This is true of soul contracts and the weaving of energy webs between us all. Some of these links we can see or feel, and some we can't.

Imagine that every meeting you have with another person or place provides a very fine ribbon, which connects from you to them. Over time, these ribbons stack up to look like thick tubes of energy.

This is often a reason why when we try to leave a relationship, home, or workplace we feel too deeply connected.

Over lifetimes, we also make sacred contracts with others, which never concluded when that lifetime ended. You can be here today in this lifetime, still in marriage, partnerships, or business contracts from many other lifetimes. When you work in an Akashic therapy session, these webs, ribbons, and cords become visible. Some are healthy, and some are not. Some cords and webs tangle us, draining our energy and life force.

Certain teachings will instruct you to cut the cords, however, I often find they are left open and raw, and then they reconnect, holding a negative energy greater than before. The only way to dissolve negative attachments is with love, forgiveness, and compassion.

A great deal of Akashic therapy works around the release and peace we make with these energies and sacred contracts. Many have made sacred contracts from lifetimes before that sabotage their spiritual path. These contracts were created when many were persecuted for their spiritual gifts or beliefs.

This will be true if you are finding challenges with working with your heart, meditation, and embracing love in your life.

Free yourself with this affirmation. Say this three times when you feel challenged to step forward with these meditations:

*I surrender all contracts I have made across
time and space that no longer serve.
I free myself of cords which
sabotage my spiritual path.
I embrace the love, light, and wisdom around me.
I bless myself and forgive my mind.
I release myself to experience new sacred
contracts of joy, peace, and happiness.*

An amazing woman crossed my path, caught in the dilemma of relationships that caused great imbalance between her new current and future life.

CASE STUDY SHANNON

I first met Amanda in Bali in May 2006, after hearing from a friend about her amazing healing abilities. After getting to know her myself, I knew that Amanda was so much more than a healer. She is a keen intuitive, a patient teacher, a great listener, and a powerful catalyst for change. This—change—is what brought Amanda and I together, for at the time of our meeting, I was saying goodbye to my beloved husband and business partner of more than eight years.

Or so I thought.

In my regular guided meditation sessions and in-depth discussions with Amanda (both of which invariably included her most trusted question: "What's the fear?"), I was able to see so much clearer just how much I was holding on to my husband, our businesses, our accomplishments, our possessions, our public personas, and the very idea of "us." I was absolutely unwilling to release him and the not-quite-yet-realized shared dreams that I saw as just beyond my grasp. Her insights put into words what I already knew in my heart: that this man and I had been deeply connected on a profound level throughout many lifetimes.

Over the course of the next two years, Amanda assisted me in what she called "cutting the cords," ties that had kept my husband and I bound for so very long. She taught me to do this with ease and grace, and today, nearly a year and a half after our divorce and the dissolution of our various business endeavors, my ex-husband and I have chosen to untie rather than cut the time-tested bonds of our shared past. We have co-created a new reality for ourselves—both individually and as people who still care a great deal for one another. I am pleased to say this reality is free from past encumbrances and drama, and abundant in unconditional love and support. For her important role in this, I will be forever grateful.

EXERCISE

Take a piece of paper and find a quiet space. Create your own sacred space and relax.

Open your divine heart and ask your heart the questions:

- What relationships do I need to release?
- What draws energy from my sacred space?
- What emotions and negative beliefs do I need to release from all my lives?

Now write down the key words and draw a heart around them.

Now sit with this list quietly and reflect.

Invite all your guides to support you and write across the paper:

> *I forgive myself, I forgive others, I ask the karmic guides to free me from the cords, ribbons, and contracts that no longer serve my higher purpose. I release the clearing to grace. I allow myself to heal and clear.*

This will allow you to start the clearing and releasing process gently and at the pace that serves you best.

I am connected to the universe.

I am a divine child of light.

I am not my story.

I learn from my story.

I am infinite.

I am manifesting something greater
in harmony with my soul.

I give thanks and gratitude for the support
and unconditional love around me.

I explore my deeper meaning of life; I delight
in the wisdom it brings to my soul.

PART THREE

Your Own Precious Akashic Journey

Opening Your Akashic Record Book

Your soul record is precious and so is the story of your life.

In previous chapters, you have worked to open your heart further, connect with your guides, and step into the etheric world that surrounds you. I invite you now to begin the process of moving through your own Akashic records.

The first time I went to work with my own Akashic record book was, in Cairo on the Giza Plateau. When I was on my third sacred journey, I visited the Sphinx and said prayers in front of the stellar (a large stone covered in hieroglyphics), which is located in the paw area. I remember feeling a sense of serenity and floating. It took me a long time to recall and ground the experience on the bus ride back to my hotel. As with many initiations, they do not appear obvious at first. The energy, I believe, lies above the crown chakra, waiting for a shift in your consciousness, at which time it can flow down through your body.

After the Sphinx visit, I returned to my room, took a shower, and fell into a deep sleep. That evening, I saw many new symbols come to me in lucid dreams. I dreamt I was back visiting the Sphinx again. I stood in front of the amazing structure and then walked around it counterclockwise. I then sat in front of the stellar and meditated. I allowed my soul to fall into the space inside the structure and wander the corridors.

In front of me, I saw tunnels of water and found myself in a small barge being sailed down the complex avenue. My ferryman I saw as Anubis, and I wore a cloak of animal print. When we reached the edge, there was a doorway, and my guide indicated for me to leave the boat and open the door. I did and entered a large room with a stone coffin, which was covered in light. In front of the coffin was a book, an old, sacred text with strange words and pictures. It was very strange, however, it all made sense. I saw this as the book of life, above and below. The above meant the heavens, and the below meant on Earth.

I placed both hands on the book and felt the golden energy trickle into and through my system, into my veins, pulsing with me.

When complete, I turned and saw my Egyptian guide; she is called Seshat, the goddess of writing. She walks beside me in all of my Egyptian journeys. Seshat is the goddess on the walls of the temples with the pointed star coming out of the top of her head. I saw her place a crystal into my heart chakra and place a star upon my head like hers. This visualization has stayed with me every day as clearly as I saw it then. I was blessed with that connection, which I know has been there many lifetimes.

That was the time when the Akashic sacred keys and codes were imprinted within my energy field. During the next few chapters, I will pass them through to you. You can then choose to open your own records, heal and clear what does not serve, and embrace the clarity that will support your spiritual journey.

You will meet some amazing guides along the way; it just requires an open heart and mind. Don't worry if you find blocks along the way. If this happens, simply return to the heart meditation and radiate your light. Do not fall into judgment, as this always closes the door to the record house. Judgment feeds the ego within us, a sad but true fact.

Practice and know that all is perfect in your divine plan. Use the release affirmation in the previous chapter.

Throughout the years, I have guided many toward their own sacred books. I will now guide you to open your own. This following meditation will open the door to your own sacred chamber. Once your book is open, you can then visit the various chambers.

The four key chambers are:
Past Lives
Present Lives
Life between Lives
Future Life

When you journey into your book, allow yourself to wander; you will feel a sense of awe and excitement. Be curious and inquisitive. Ask the book questions. Your guides may appear to show and help you. This will be a stage when your Crown chakra really engages with the other dimensions and your dreams may become more lucid and your clairvoyant sight increases. Remember, you are in control of this whole journey and will only go to places for your highest good.

Opening the Akashic record book Meditation

Find yourself a quiet space and have your journal ready.
Ensure you have a sacred energy around you that brings clarity and safety.

Take a few deep breaths and relax
and begin the meditation.
Now we begin, to open your Akashic record book.

Relax and allow your attention to wander to your heart.
Imagine a bright light growing in your heart
and spreading throughout your body.
See the light move down your lower body and
down through your legs, through your feet and
like tree roots all the way into the earth.
See your roots of shining light reach
the crystal of Gaia and connect.
As you do you, see the crystal sparkle and the

light rise back up though the roots into your
feet, legs, and body, back to the heart.
See the light rise from your heart and move
through your throat into your head, and like a
fountain, allow it to move up through your head
into the sky and connect with a star above.
See the light move back to you until the pulse
remains in your heart and the light, which
surrounds you, is a column from sky to earth.
Now focus on your heart and let's warm it awake.
Imagine it has a glowing star with five points.
To open all the points, allow the heart energy to flow and
focus on the happiest moments or people in your life.
Relax and smile, and let the happy
thoughts expand this heart chakra.
Send light around this star.
Feel your shoulders relax back, and
feel the peace around you.
Now see a small flame in the center of the star.
Allow yourself to flow into the flame.
This is the flame of transformation and transmutation;
it clears negativity and brings purification and clarity.
Warm yourself in the flame and smile.
Now look down and see a pearl, a beautiful,
translucent, and radiant pearl.
Hold it in your hand, gently send it love,
and be amazed at how beautiful it is.
This is your heart, beloved, your divine heart,
The perfect essence of yourself when
you were created as a star seed.

And this is now the place you can visit and ask your truth.
You are connected to the earth and
universe and in your divine heart.
Now is the time to open your sacred Akashic record book.

Imagine you're walking into a room, a
library; there is a chair and table.
The floor will be two colors of tiles.
There will be lights.
Notice the other things around your room.
See the décor and relax as your attention
wanders around this space.
Walk over to the desk.
On the desk, watch as a large book
appears in front of you.
Look at the color of the book.
Feel how old the book is.
Beam a stream of light from your
heart onto the book cover.
See the book come to life, notice the
colors, symbols, and words.
See yourself place your left hand on the cover.
Allow your heart energy to flow to the
cover and unlock the records.
See the book open and the pictures or
messages connect with your awareness.
Stay with this book until you feel ready to move on.
When ready, close the book and place
your right hand on the cover.

See the color fade, and allow yourself to return
to your reality refreshed and radiant.

Now take a few moments to write down your experience.

- Describe your room.
- What did the book look like?
- Can you draw the symbols?
- What words appeared?
- What messages came forward?
- What did you discover about yourself?

We all find different images and messages. The majority are of hope, direction, and clarity. Sometimes, however, darker images appear. This can often stop the process as the client returns to fear.

I was trained in the Egyptian and Mayan traditions that embrace the light and observe the darkness. Often we must journey through both. If you do find yourself in fear, it's very simple. Breathe and illuminate your heart.

Make the statement, "Angels, come to me now; Archangel Michael, protect me now."

Say it in your head or out loud, and repeat over and over again until the fear subsides.

Now that we have journeyed through the various stages to gather your keys and codes to the Akashic map, the time has come to bring them all together.

The key meditations you have worked with are:
Divine Heart—To connect you to the higher dimensions (used in all the Akashic sessions).

The Sanctuary—To create sacred space to work with your guides.

Opening the Akashic Book—To access the records to heal,

clear, and gain clarity on your spiritual path (used in all the Akashic sessions).

We now work with this as building blocks to journey through the records. These will be integral parts of each meditation.

Don't worry, I have taken the time to build each meditation in a way that flows easily for you. You can record the meditation yourself or work with another person. I often find just sitting with this book and gently reading the meditation, you see images or messages occur.

You can decide which area of the record houses you wish to go to. I would suggest you work with the past and then the present. After this, examine your life between lives, and finally your future. This helps keep the timeline fluid.

Remember to focus on your perfect intention and move forward with ease and grace.

PAST LIVES WITH AKASHIC THERAPY

As energy souls, we have incarnated many times—a cycle that has continued for each soul since it was first created into an earthbound form. Over those lives, each soul has endured both positive and negative life experiences. If you can, imagine that in this timeline, the soul can store this trauma at a deep cellular level. The Akashic works in the realms of past lives to clear and heal karma from previous incarnations. This karmic trauma is recorded in the Akashic books and shown back to us in the form of past-life visualizations.

Akashic therapy goes into that record and highlights the unresolved issue or pain. Then it places forgiveness, peace, love, and compassion into the event.

Although the historic event or record cannot be altered, the emotional and spiritual response to the event can be healed and re-evaluated or redefined.

In past lives, I find people are layered with past-life karma and sacred contracts to places and people. These connections can lie dormant for lifetimes until the soul is ready to release them.

I do meet people who claim to have "cleared" all their karma and past lives. This is true of the karma, however, records cannot be erased. Others may have been involved in that event who have not given their free will and choice for rewrites.

Each of us is responsible for our own Akashic work. We heal our energy, and it will have an impact on others involved. However, it is their choice whether to mirror the healing and reflect it back.

Imagine a large highway with holes and cracks; the

highway stretches behind you and in front of you. Sometimes the cracks start far back, and although they are thinner around you this lifetime, they are still there to cause challenge within this lifetime. By going back to the original record, you can go back to the initial point of impact. Here you can fill over and heal the damage or claim forgiveness with the person with whom you caused the crack. At this point, you often understand why the event happened and its purpose for your and another's soul journey.

We also must remember that we have all committed deeds and actions that have been distressing to others in past lives. I first discovered this when I looked at my own records; I was on an angel workshop, content to know I was full of love and light and working in the angelic method of blessings and kindness.

My personal learning was tested when I began having flashbacks of another time around the Tudors in England. My teacher offered to work through a past life with me and we went back to a time in Glastonbury when there had been great suffering and darkness around the area. I saw the choices I had made in that time and it was very sobering and challenging for my ego to know that this had occurred. I went into a deep place of forgiveness and compassion and the tears flowed. When the session was over my teacher and I were both a little stunned and shaken. Tea and biscuits was the order of the day. It now made sense why I was drawn to this location and always held myself in my best energy. Heart space was a contract and lesson I had regarding this lifetime and events. I also lost my sense of judgment for others and myself. Who was I now to judge poor choices and damage caused to others? Which is why I can offer this as session work. I'm not shocked or disturbed by the shadows and stories others bring for I've seen the shadow side of myself and leant to accept that and love that for what it was and when it was.

Often, those who have harmed us are repaying karma for their actions. Until healing occurs, the cycle of harm and distress continues.

What is remarkable is that karmic clearing and healing can be completed by an individual alone toward some other person in their life. The other people will have no idea on a physical level, except that something has healed or feels lighter around them or regarding a situation.

Connections to Places on the Planet

Akashic past life shows us why we are connected and contracted to certain places. While working in sacred sites and temples, I noticed that the guides and guardians and even the traders appeared to have been bound to these sites for lifetimes. It is always wise to pay respect and attention to these special souls. I had revelations regarding this and past-life connections.

The first was in the sacred Mayan ruins in Copan, Honduras. This is simply one of the most exquisite temple sites for beauty and energy I have had the honor to work in. The first time I stepped into the site, amazing things happened, and I gained greater clairvoyance. On my first trip to the Copan site, I had the gift of a shaman tour guide with me. As we entered the site, he began to race across the grass (which I thought was strange). He picked up a macaw feather and handed it to me. At the time, I did not realize how rare and sacred this was. All of the guides have these feathers on their guiding sticks to teach their groups ancient knowledge. The feathers are orange and bright on one side and dark purple-blue on the other. The guides believed that Mayan life was ruled "as above and below in balance," and shadow (the purple side) follows into light (the orange side). I was deeply honored that day. I realized that many lifetimes before, I had led ceremony here, and this feather was a sign to tell me the energy was still with me. I use the feather in blessings and ceremonies to gain clarity.

On that trip, I gained further insight to the guardians of such places. One evening, my friend and I were talking to a few local guides who had been born into the town. We asked if they ever wanted to leave "No, we are bound to this place," they replied.

I thought this bizarre at the time, but on reading the records, I found that it is true. Certain shamans have chosen to be guardians of these sites through lifetimes until the sacred sites require them no more. They know the secrets, as I explored further, I confirmed my theory in the Dendara temple in Egypt.

I was visiting Dendara in 2006 and I sought a quiet space to reflect. I wandered down to the left-hand front corner and marveled at the beautiful Hathors face in the ceiling. I saw a guard step out from behind one of the columns, wearing a long Egyptian robe dress and turban. I hoped he worked in the temple, but then again nothing surprises me in temples anymore.

I indicated I just wished to sit a little and meditate. He beckoned to me and pointed to a stone, which held a plastic bag in place. He lifted the stone and bag and pointed for me to sit. I checked around and found myself very much alone. It was mid-afternoon, and I was glad for the shade and rest.

But then I questioned whether it was safe for me to sit in the dust, far away from others. *No,* I thought, *time to stop the chatter and embrace the experience.*

I smiled at the guardian and bowed my head; then he moved to the side and stood with his back to me, as if holding and guarding space. I sat down on the spot and waited.

I closed my eyes and connected with the face above; at once a column of light came down and surrounded me. I dared not open my eyes. I felt in a total space of peace and joy; it moved through every cell in my body like an initiation. My spine tingled, and I felt a wave of energy. After a while, I was finished. I stood and grounded myself. The guardian turned to me and smiled, and we both bowed with hands in prayer. I gave my little financial exchange; he nodded and replaced the plastic bag and stone over the area where I had been sitting. Wow, who would have thought such a humble space could be so sacred!

Past-life Akashic therapy can uncover many messages.

Serena has been on her spiritual path for a many years. She attends meditation and healing groups and has traveled to Egypt. I held a video Skype session with her for clarity of messages from her guides and the universe. We went very gently into the divine heart meditation. With Akashic work, the messages can come before or after the session. They all filter at their own pace; her eyes gently closed at the sound of my voice, and we went first into the garden sanctuary. I asked the colors of her butterflies, and they were orange. So I'm noting that the transformation has to do with the sacral area. Her flowers are pink blooms, so I'm recognizing she needs to feel support. We wait a little while in the garden as her guide approaches. I watch her body relax further as she has her conversation with him and he gives her the gift of "grace." We then move her toward the door at the end of the garden. I ask her to open it with her left hand, and she pauses at the doorway, hesitant. She tells me she wants to re-center her energy and just gather her thoughts, and I ask her to focus on her intention at this point. When she is ready to proceed, she tells me she is in a path of light, all golden with golden paths here and there, and she is a little confused which path to take. This is perfect. I tell her, "Walk a little; you are on the matrix of light. The universal gird, which connects the energy of everything. The door will appear when you are ready. And of course it did. Again I asked her to open it with her left hand; this time was easy, and she found herself in a meadow area next to some woods with trees. This felt like the earth plane to her, but Serena felt uneasy. She was searching for something or someone. I was aware that whatever she was searching for was in the woods, and it felt animal, mainly doglike. I asked her to sit and just watch it show itself. I waited as she said, "It's a wolf, a really large and strong one." I asked what it was doing.

"It's carrying something in its mouth," and her emotion began to shake. "It's a small child," I said. "Yes, my baby," she replied. "Has the baby died?" I asked. "Yes," she whimpered. "Okay, well allow the wolf to settle, and we stay calm." I then asked a strange question; I asked whom her conflict of care was for. I saw her care and have love for the child but also for the wolf. A great compassion for them both.

I guided her to focus on the baby soul coming toward her, a beautiful, shining bright light, full of giggles and mischief. She did, and she held the energy close before we moved it to the universal light. Before the soul left, it told her that it had been searching for adventure, and it had been its time to leave. We watched the butterflies float away with the little soul. I brought her focus back to the wolf. I asked her to ask the wolf for its message. It was simple:

"This is life, this is nature, and it's not personal."

She made her peace with the wolf and we set off to return.

It was an interesting session, because I told her we were ready to leave and she should come back through the door and close and seal it with her right hand. Just as I was going to lead her back through the golden matrix, I lost the video connection. Okay, I thought, all is in divine order. I quickly Skyped directions and waited. A few minutes later, the line came back. She told me she had waited and called her angels and created affirmations. All was safe, well, and perfect. I quickly moved her through the next door, closed it with the right hand, exiting through the garden. We thanked the guide who had waited and then returned back to the third dimensional space, disconnecting the golden cords above and below.

She was delighted; she had had this memory of a lost child soul around her for a while and had been unable to gather the message. Now a very happy lady who had gained clarity about nature and the questions she had on life.

For me, I learned that holding space is perfect, but with simple instructions and good intentions, you can follow simple directions to your own Akashic work. It does not need a full OBE (out-of-body experience). Simple information can be gathered in those gentle meditation moments of the day.

Past Life Meditations

There are two sessions in Akashic therapy that work extremely well with past lives.

The first one is a short meditation to locate the key areas around the globe where you have had significant past lives; the other is the past-life journey meditation.

How to find significant places around the globe; this can also be used on the universe to include star systems and planets.

Find your quiet sacred space, and open your journal. You could draw or print a map of the world, if you are able.

Now go into your heart space and expand
the light within your heart.
Relax and take a few deep breaths.
See the bright, radiant light from your heart
reach down to the center of the Earth.
See the column of light spring back from the
Earth center through you and up to the sky.

Feel connected and at peace with all around you.
Ask gently for your spiritual guides and angels to
help you connect to your Akashic records.
Relax and allow your awareness just to
wander to another dimension.
Now ask the Akashic records to show
you a globe of planet Earth.
Ask the globe to spin in front of you.
See the globe stop; lights will appear on
the countries that you connect with.
Look closer; names of cities may appear.
Once you are ready, thank your guides
and return to your present space.
Allow the cords above and below you to release and
bring happiness and healing back to your heart.

When you feel ready, write down the places that come to you.

- Which countries stepped forward?
- Which cities came to mind?
- Did you recall anything else?
- Did these places bring you fear?

Take a moment to review your list.

Sometimes ancient areas such as Atlantis or Lemuria come to mind. They are not on the physical map at the moment, but their energy remains.

You can use this list to clear the energy without actually visiting; just write the name and location down and surround it with a heart symbol. This will start the healing process.

You can, of course, use the next past-life meditation to visit these countries for further clarity.

Now we can work through the second exercise and visit a past life in the Akashic.

Find yourself a quiet space and have your journal ready.
Ensure you have a sacred energy around you that brings clarity and safety.
Take a few deep breaths and relax and begin the meditation.
Now we begin to open your Akashic past life record book.

Relax and allow your attention to wander to your heart.

Imagine a bright light growing in your heart
and spreading throughout your body.
See the light move down your lower body and
down through your legs, through your feet, and
like tree roots all the way into the earth.
See your roots of shining light reach
the crystal of Gaia and connect.
As you do, you see the crystal sparkle and the
light rise back up though the roots into your
feet, legs, and body, back to the heart.
See the light rise from your heart and move
through your throat into your head. Like a
fountain, allow it to move up through your head
into the sky and connect with a star above.
See the light move back to you, until the pulse
remains in your heart and the light that surrounds
you is a column from sky to earth.
Now focus on your heart and let's warm it awake.
Imagine it has a glowing star with five points.

To open all the points, allow the heart energy to flow and
focus on the happiest moments or people in your life.
Relax and smile, and let the happy
thoughts expand this heart chakra.
Send light around this star.
Feel your shoulders relax back, and
feel the peace around you.
Now see a small flame in the center of the star.
Allow yourself to flow into the flame.
This is the flame of transformation and transmutation;
it clears negativity and brings purification and clarity.
Warm yourself in the flame and smile.
Now look down and see a pearl, a beautiful
translucent and radiant pearl.
Hold it in your hand, gently send it love,
and be amazed at how beautiful it is.
This is your heart, beloved, your divine heart,
the perfect essence of yourself when
you were created as a star seed.
And this is now the place you can visit and ask your truth.
You are connected to the earth and
universe and in your divine heart.
Now is the time to open your sacred Akashic record book.

Imagine yourself back in your library room.
Are any of your guides with you?
See your book on the desk, and open it with
your left hand. See it glow with golden light.
Then see a doorway appear in the room,
with golden light shining behind it.

Move toward this door.
Open the door gently and step forward.
Step into the lifetime of the past and look around.
What does the environment look like?
Who is with you?
How do you feel?
What is happening?
What have you returned to this Akashic record
to heal, clear, and gain clarity with?
What action do you need to take?
Who and what do you need to forgive?
What high-vibration lesson do you need to
know and return back to this lifetime with?
Just keep breathing and smile light energy into your heart.
Send love into this story.
Do you have any contracts to end?
Do you see the scrolls?
Do you have any cords to cut?
See the cords turn to ribbons and fold up and dissolve?
Allow your higher spirit guides to step
forward to help you with this.
When ready, see the door again in front of you.
Go back through the door.
Close the door.
Stand back in your library.
Close your Akashic record book.
See your guides.
Smile, and if you need to, take time to rest.
See butterflies and radiant light around you.
When ready, return to your space, see the light

disconnect from above and below, and create
an amazing feeling of joy in your heart.
Ground yourself and know you have
achieved a healing clearing and clarity.
If tears flow, let them.
Relax and take time in this sacred heart space of love.

Now take a moment to write the key points from your experience.

- What did you see?
- Who was there with you?
- What did you feel?
- What did you heal?
- What did you learn?
- Was this past-life karma playing through this lifetime?

Now release this past life; let it go with love and light.

Present Life with Akashic Therapy

New issues, current karma, and life lessons can create learning within present lives. When we become so involved in the day-to-day issues, we are unable to see past the underlying spiritual message. Akashic therapy allows you to hover above the emotional storyline veils, to understand and comprehend the truth at a deeper level. When healing and clearing relationships, I suggest new, positive contracts be placed into the Akashic record, to allow the healing and clarity to continue.

There are three key areas that Akashic Therapy works with in present lives:

Intimate Relationships

Letting go of relationships that no longer serve; healing relationships; attracting new and beautiful relationships into your life.

Abundance and Success

Attracting abundance of wealth, experiences, and happiness in life; creating purposeful success in the life and career you choose.

Property and Living Conditions

Releasing homes and property that no longer serve; attracting positive living environments that bring joy and peace into your life.

This chapter will explore the key areas and then lead a meditation into the Akashic sanctuary, where you can work on one, two, or all three of these areas of your present life.

Intimate Relationships

Many of us attract partners into our lives, and the attractions are unexplainable. We meet them, and in an instant, we know the connection is very strong. Many call this a soul mate.

The term *soul mate* is very confusing, especially when the relationship hits troubled times or has actually fulfilled its contract. We can often hang on to the person because we believe nothing can replace him or her, even if this union is a destructible one. At the same time, you may hold a soul so dear, your heart leaps at the sound of his or her name. However, they may not be ready to embrace that. I often see this with clients, where one holds ribbons out to connect and the other person I clairvoyantly see is turning his or her back. The answer is simple: move on; you cannot spin a web around anyone's heart. You can lure and entice, in the end, the cords will suffocate you.

When working with people's records, it is my understanding that we have a soul group, a group of energy cells or people who incarnate around us in certain lifetimes or choose to watch over us from the life-between-life platforms. A twin flame, I find from readings, happens when a person's energy splits in previous lives and they become like two peas from a pod.

Each soul group will have a mixture of personalities, and when a personality from one soul group meets the same type of personality from another soul group, they think, *hey, they are the same as me,* and therefore the confusion begins.

Cords and contracts are exchanged and vows made in the present lifetime, which can contradict the cords and contracts from karmic previous lifetimes.

You see how messy and confusing this can be.

Akashic work allows you to see the individual for who and what they are for you, without the story and emotional ego. Once you see this and look at why this person is in your life, you can then decide how you wish to pursue the matters of your heart.

CASE STUDY—KAREN

One amazing woman I worked with struggled to let go of her relationship with her husband, even though they were in a divorce proceeding and we knew he was never going to return to her. I took her into a present-day meditation, into the sanctuary garden, and with the help of her guides, she saw her husband sit in front of her. As she sits in front of him, I help her feel her guides around her for support. I then have her tell him how she felt and then be silent while he responds. Working from the heart space can produce the most gentle of responses, even when the message is not what you wish to hear. She told me how he told her it was over and it was time to move on. I asked her to work with words of forgiveness for him and her, and that now it was time to release the contracts and cords.

I had her imagine a red ribbon tied with a bow around them both. I asked her to undo the ribbons, which each held around the other and then to fold them gently and return the ribbons. As she did this, tears flowed onto her face, but not once did she sob or cry out loud. These tears were the emotions leaving her. I allowed them to hug and then for him to go. Her guides placed her ribbon under a tree for safekeeping until she wished to use it again. They divorced with ease, and when things became challenging, she would go to this place of serenity and peace and send love to the situation. And after time spent healing, she found a relationship that fulfils her even greater than the one before.

A few words of caution with past-life relationship episodes: Sometimes people from past lives re-enter and try to relive the relationship in this present time. It is very important to be cautious and not let that path follow again. This is a lifetime to be enjoyed for *this* lifetime of experience. While it is important to work through the karma and connections, it can be confusing to overlap for nostalgia, reconnecting romantically this present lifetime because you shared a past life.

In past lives, we chose roles to play, but they may not be the roles appropriate for this lifetime.

So when someone says to you, "Have we met in a previous lifetime? I'm feeling a connection. Were we lovers?" **be warned and beware**.

Abundance and Success

This is a material world, and we often measure our success by the wealth we have or had in previous lifetimes. We can often reminisce for a time when life was opulent and we wanted for nothing. Money, power, and greed bring some of the biggest and most painful lessons for people.

This world has an abundance of life, but when we only see the money sign, we deny ourselves all the other amazing opportunities of life. Akashic therapy allows you to see the energy around you with your abundance and success stream. You can see if it's flowing or if it's blocked.

When I'm working with business owners, I will take them to the energy or colors aligned with the business through meditation. They will often observe single colors such as red and not the full spectrum. When this is the case, it shows me that there is a lack of rainbow flow, which works with the universe. Rainbow light fuses to produce brilliant light, and that is why I believe some businesses and financial portfolios shine and some lack luster. When a business is grounded only in red chakra energy, I would predict this business would race to success and then fall at the first recession. I would encourage this business to look at their triple bottom line, to include profits, people, and the planet.

If the energy is confused and the emotional feel of the

business is in panic, we often see yellows; but dark gray shades which mean the business is lost in flow and true identity. I usually find the business is not paying bills and living off of sales targets and not profits.

Usually, a present-life Akashic session helps to heal this. I take clients back where they can examine the lessons and contracts they wish to learn in this lifetime. They understand why the money comes and goes the way it does. Once the lesson is understood, the fight is often over, and they can change their relationship to a more positive one.

Property and Living Conditions

I have many requests from clients to help them sell their properties or leave a location in life that no longer serves them.

In Akashic therapy, we visualize the current living location and the sacred contracts and cords surrounding it. Very often, we are held in a certain location until we clear our karma or learn a life lesson. You can make peace with these locations and visualize packing everything into boxes ready to leave.

This is a powerful affirmation I use with clients when they feel clear and ready to move on:

I am moving.
I am releasing the space and place
which no longer serves.
I'm am asking my guides to support my journey
with grace and ease to somewhere new which
serves my highest good and well-being.
I am packing my energy and worldly
goods into boxes to take with me.
I am ending my contracts with (the location
address) and setting it free from me.
I ask the Akashic to hold this affirmation
with the energy of love and peace.
And so it is.

Present life Meditation

Before you start, think of which area you wish to examine and work with.

Find yourself a quiet space and have your journal ready.

Ensure you have a sacred energy around you that brings clarity and safety.

Take a few deep breaths and relax
and begin the meditation.
Now we begin, to open your Akashic record book.

Relax and allow your attention to wander to your heart.
Imagine a bright light growing in your heart
and spreading throughout your body.
See the light move down you lower body and
down through your legs, through your feet, and
like tree roots all the way into the earth.
See your roots of shining light reach
the crystal of Gaia and connect.
As you do, you see the crystal sparkle and the
light rise back up through the roots into your
feet, legs, and body, back to the heart.
See the light rise from your heart and move
through your throat into your head. Like a
fountain, allow it to move up through your head
into the sky and connect with a star above.
See the light move back to you until the pulse
remains in your heart and the light that surrounds
you is a column from sky to earth.
Now focus on your heart and let's warm it awake.

Imagine it has a glowing star with five points.
To open all the points, allow the heart energy to flow and
focus on the happiest moments or people in your life.
Relax and smile and let the happy
thoughts expand this heart chakra.
Send light around this star.
Feel your shoulders relax back, and
feel the peace around you.
Now see a small flame in the center of the star.
Allow yourself to flow into the flame.
This is the flame of transformation and transmutation;
it clears negativity and brings purification and clarity.
Warm yourself in the flame and smile.
Now look down and see a pearl, a beautiful,
translucent, and radiant pearl.
Hold it in your hand, gently send it love,
and be amazed at how beautiful it is.
This is your heart, beloved, your divine heart,
the perfect essence of yourself when
you were created as a star seed.
And this is now the place you can visit and ask your truth.
You are connected to the earth and
universe and in your divine heart.
Now is the time to open your sacred Akashic record book.

Imagine yourself back in your library room.
Are any of your guides with you?

See your book on the desk, and open it with
your left hand. See it glow with golden light.
Then see a doorway appear in the room
with golden light shining behind it.
Move toward this door.
Open the door gently and step forward.
Imagine you are in a garden sanctuary.
What are the flowers like? What color are the butterflies?
Take time to look around your
sanctuary, breathe, and be safe.

Now look across the garden and see a
beautiful light coming toward you.
This is your gatekeeper to your records
and a guardian for you.
Take time to connect with this guide.
Ask their messages.
Receive their gifts.
What does the environment look like?
Who is with you?
Observe the seating areas around the garden and wander
over to see the souls with whom you can connect.
How do you feel?
What is happening?
What have you returned to this Akashic sanctuary
to heal, clear, and gain clarity with?
What action do you need to take?
Who and what do you need to forgive?
It may be others; it may be yourself.

Now create a circle of roses. Imagine the color
and fragrance that resonates with you.
See two chairs, one for you and one for
the person you seek healing with.
Speak the words and send love and listen.
Hear the words from their heart whisper the truth.
Breathe and clear any ribbons or cords that do not serve.
Let the situation go, and continue
to walk into your garden.
See the board on the wall and the words
that describe your present life.
How do you feel about them?
Do you wish to change anything?
Write with love and peace in your heart.
What high-vibration lesson do you need to
know and return back to this lifetime with?
See golden leaves of abundance swirling around you.
Just keep breathing and smile light energy into your heart.
Send love into this story.
Allow your higher spirit guides to step
forward, to help you with this.

When ready, see the door again in front of you.
Go back through the door.
Close the door.
Stand back in your library.
Close your Akashic record book.
See your guides.
When ready, return to your space, see the light

disconnect from above and below, and create
an amazing feeling of joy in your heart.
Ground yourself and know you have achieved
a healing, clearing, and clarity.
If tears flow, let them.
Relax and take time in this sacred heart space of love.

Now take a moment to write the key points from your experience.

- What did you see?
- Who was there with you?
- What did you feel?
- What did you heal?
- What did you learn?
- What did you release and clear?
- What did you embrace within your present life?
- What clarity did you gain?

LIFE BETWEEN LIVES

If we imagine that we are made from energy, our soul is the energy life pulse switch. When our physical body dies, this energy switch leaves and like a magnet flows back to the central source.

This space is known as the area where souls recycle themselves. Knowing this creates great comfort, understanding that we all go somewhere when we pass on from this world.

You go to an area in which the soul creates the life lessons, contracts, and karma that you will have in the next lifetime.

You can visit this space in order to make sense of your roles upon the Earth and within the universe. Currently, when souls return to Earth, they typically forget previous lives, although some remember. For me, simply knowing that these records exist and having the recall is my awakening to a new consciousness. Now with the advances in spiritual teachings, more people are remembering their truth and how amazing the universe is and the energies all around.

My first life-between-lives session as a student was incredible. This was a time in life when I was taking any spiritual experience I could and devouring the information and teaching. I went along to the session and found myself totally at ease. The session, used hypnotherapy. Now with the divine heart meditation and Akashic therapy, the method is quicker and easier.

In my session with a gifted therapist named Kate, we went through the countdown stage and mental cool-down. By allowing my thoughts to fade, I found myself drifting through the guided visualization.

To my surprise, I found myself in a room, which looked like an amphitheatre. I was in front of three large TV screens. I was wearing a gown of shimmering white, all around me was clean and clear, but very nondescript. I started seeing images on the screen.

Kate began to question what I was viewing on the screens.

"Well, I'm seeing myself on the last Egypt trip. I'm talking and teaching a small group outside the pyramids on Giza," I said.

But then, suddenly I was seeing myself on the second and third screen like a video playback. This was one event with three versions: my version, the student version, and the cosmic version. This was truly a moment to stop for reflection. I realized that when we move from this earthbound space to that of another dimension, the realties are all apparent.

I could see the areas where I could have slowed the pace of discussion, and also where to show compassion. This made me think very carefully later on with my teachings, because the review in this life zone will be from many viewpoints.

Kate very skillfully moved me through the journey and away from the screen. I could have been happy to stay with this viewing all day. But now it was time to flow through to the next stage. We came to a steel gate, and from nowhere, I saw Kate in spirit beside me. This was a little surprising, as it did not look like her, but at the same time, it felt like her. The door opened, and I moved forward and saw my version of the Akashic library. The walls were dark oak-paneled and the floor black-and-white checked. Candles lit the area all around. Books were on the table, but I did not dare read. For some reason at this point, I felt I did not have the access codes for these publications; they did not belong to me.

I wandered a little around this area and felt Kate growing a little impatient with me. I decided it was time to return to my world and indicated that I had had enough time in session. I returned still with the vivid vision and feeling of this space and place, and I asked Kate how she was feeling. "Well, you know when you went into the library and through the gate?" she said.

"Yes," I replied.

"Well, I had a flashback," she admitted.

This can sometimes happen; you can find yourself linked with a client in a karmic way.

"Well," she said, "it all has to do with our first meeting, when I felt uncomfortable around you."

"Go on," I prompted.

Oh, please don't say she's going to say I burnt the library or worse, I'm thinking.

She continued further that she knew her job was to collect the records from souls who have come into this place to review their journeys with their guides. She explained that she collected the records, brought them to me, and handed them through the gates.

"And you would sit there at that big, grand desk and check them, and then, lady!" she said. I could feel a rising in her tone. "You send them back and ask for further clarity, detail, and intention setting for the next life!" Her voice was shrill and high with emotion.

"Do you know how many we get through some days?" she wailed. "But no, it's always more detail, more healing," she continued. "I think I came down here for a rest, and here you are again, making me work."

We both were silent for a moment, and I looked at her. "I'm so sorry, so sorry," I whispered.

I asked forgiveness, and we laughed the way women do when they feel supported and genuine sister love.

"I'll be more patient next time, I promise," I said.

It was a big wake-up call and a fabulous realization of the role my soul has to play in the bigger picture of life.

CASE STUDY—GEORGE

While working on a male client, George, we were looking at his life patterns with power, greed, and ego. His life had been very successful in the business world, yet every decade, it appeared he would nearly lose it all and have to struggle back through the pattern of massive action and chaos relationships. As this had now happened three times in his current life, he was keen to change the direction. At first, we looked at past lives, but nothing appeared to be significant to this particular cycle. There were many years spent as a warrior; we went through some amazing voyages to Rome, Greece, and the pirates around the Caribbean. Still the common thread or lesson evaded us.

On his next session, we agreed to go to the life between lives and read the scrolls or witness the three screens. George was skeptical about fluffy clouds; however, he followed the plan. We went through his garden of sanctuary and floated on the cloud till we reached his gateway. His guide, whom we had met in sessions before, met him.

We first went to look at the TV screens. True to form, a scene of a battle and an army of men played around. I guided him to pay particular attention to the screen from which the cosmic viewing was taking place. We could see and feel the passion on the soldiers' faces, the relief when they fell; we watched their souls rise out of their bodies. The guide appeared beside us, and I asked who was the other figure that had stepped forward. George replied, "Michael." At that point, I saw the message.

George worked in the Archangel Michael department for protection and support of warriors on the Earth plane. George described the viewing further and then said something interesting; he began to talk of "honor contract codes," how the karmic path of a warrior was to win victory or die on the field.

This lesson for George, I felt, was the key and the missing link. We stayed in this zone, and I relaxed George further, and we placed his contract scroll in front of him. I also asked Archangel Michael to explain what it meant to be a warrior for spirit and heart. George heard his message that had been tangled in the loop for many lifetimes. George had originally had a contract of honor and to support warriors; however, many lifetimes of battles and killing had led to a buildup of karma, which rolled from one life to the next, never clearing. George's heart told him he would be safe and to trust; that was why the recurring conflict and near loss of business played out: George was testing his role. It was not until the loss became critical that George would turn to spirit and ask for help.

I then asked George to rewrite the contract and to create clarity with love, honor, and healing. We thanked his guides and returned to this lifetime.

George felt lighter and, as he explained it, free. He had created chaos with relationships, forcing others to fight for contracts and then be ungraciously dismissed when they failed. He saw and felt a new clear relationship with contract, and we laughed as we imagined how long he had been running this timeline.

Life between lives Meditation

Find yourself a quiet space and have your journal ready.

Ensure you have a sacred energy around you that brings clarity and safety.

Take a few deep breaths and relax and begin the meditation.

Now we begin, to open your Akashic
life between life record book.

Relax and allow your attention to wander to your heart.
Imagine a bright light growing in your heart
and spreading throughout your body.
See the light move down your lower body and
down through your legs, through your feet, and
like tree roots all the way into the earth.
See your roots of shining light reach
the crystal of Gaia and connect.
As you do, you see the crystal sparkle and the
light rise back up though the roots into your
feet, legs, and body, back to the heart.
See the light rise from your heart and move
through your throat into your head. Like a
fountain, allow it to move up through your head
into the sky and connect with a star above.
See the light move back to you until the pulse
remains in your heart and the light, which
surrounds you, is a column from sky to earth.
Now focus on your heart and let's warm it awake.
Imagine it has a glowing star with five points.

To open all the points, allow the heart energy to flow and
focus on the happiest moments or people in your life.
Relax and smile and let the happy
thoughts expand this heart chakra.
Send light around this star.
Feel your shoulders relax back, and
feel the peace around you.
Now see a small flame in the center of the star.
Allow yourself to flow into the flame.
This is the flame of transformation and transmutation;
it clears negativity and brings purification and clarity.
Warm yourself in the flame and smile.
Now look down and see a pearl, a beautiful,
translucent, and radiant pearl.
Hold it in your hand, gently send it love,
and be amazed at how beautiful it is.
This is your heart, beloved, your divine heart,
the perfect essence of yourself when
you were created as a star seed.
And this is now the place you can visit and ask your truth.
You are connected to the Earth and
universe and in your divine heart.
Now is the time to open your sacred Akashic record book.
Ask to go to the area of lives between lives.
Ask that you be able to access the knowledge
and truth beyond the dimensions.
Imagine yourself back in your library room.
Are any of your guides with you?

See your book on the desk and open it with
your left hand; see it glow with golden light.
Then see a doorway appear in the room
with golden light shining behind it.
Move toward this door.
Open the door gently and step forward.
When you feel ready, look across and see clouds arrive.
Walk toward the cloud of choice.
Imagine just floating up.
As you reach the blue sky, you will see
other clouds form to make a bridge.
Walk across this bridge.
See the gate with your name across it.
As you reach it, hold the space and see the handle;
reach with your left hand and open the door.
Step into the life-between-life world and look around.
What does the environment look like?
Who is with you?
How do you feel?
What is happening?
What have you returned to this Akashic
record to gain clarity with?
What is your role here?
What is your job and purpose?
Whom do you watch over on Earth from this place?
Now turn and see the screening room.
Take time in front of your three video screens.
What images do you see?

What are key lessons on the contracts
you have in this life to learn?
What action do you need to take?
Who and what do you need to forgive?
What high-vibration lesson do you need to
know and return back to this lifetime with?
Just keep breathing and smile light energy into your heart.
Send love into this story.

When ready, see the door again in front of you.
Go back through the door.
Close the door.
Stand back in your library.
Close your Akashic record book.
See your guides.
When ready, return to your space, see the light
disconnect from above and below, and create
an amazing feeling of joy in your heart.
Ground yourself and know you have achieved
a healing, clearing, and clarity.
If tears flow, let them.
Relax and take time in this sacred heart space of love.

Now take a moment to write the key points from your experience.

- What did you see?
- Who was there with you?
- What was your purpose, role, or job?
- Whom do you watch over?

- What did you feel?
- What did you heal?
- What did you learn and discover about yourself?
- What did you release and clear?
- What clarity did you gain?
- What did you find and discover about divine purpose?

The Future through Akashic Therapy

We are all aware that time will advance in some way, and many are keen to know what the future holds. Akashic work can visit two aspects of timelines in the future.

The first is within the present life. Akashic therapy can indicate a timeline of lessons, spiritual teachers, and guides. You can move toward the future knowing the manifestation for life you have created or projected. You can then choose to make changes or know that they are maintaining a flow of joy and peace.

The second is where you can travel into future lifetimes and see amazing moments of joyful living or destruction. This prompts action within you and can open your consciousness to a greater responsibility of care in this life.

After many trips to Egypt, my peer group had worked through their past lives. My work began to alter, and many clients came seeking future guidance.

They wished to know who their guides were and how far they were on their path of initiation and ascension.

Case study—Nigel

There was one dear friend who traveled many times to Egypt and now takes groups to Nepal and the Himalayas. He is a beautiful soul and actually has the look and glow of a modern-day Buddha. He spent his first few Egypt trips working though karma with others and gaining his personal empowerment. His life was balanced, and he had a great job. But there was something more he felt was needed in his life. He came to me one day to ask if I could move forward on the timeline to a future life or the future in his life.

I was trained in remote viewing, so I understood that time is just like a ladder you can go up and down to gain information. Therefore I agreed if the Akashic had information regarding the past and present, then perhaps it had insight for myself and him going forward.

We went into the divine heart and cleared a little karmic issue that was there. Then, rather than taking him though the library doorway, we went into an elevator.

It was bright and shining, and inside he had over a hundred floors to choose from. (I later realized these were dimensions.) He chose the floor, and we nervously waited for the elevator door to re-open. When it did, I was taken aback. I saw an old Chinese man in amazing robes of red. Nigel smiled and began describing a Chinese wise holy man. He then stepped out from the elevator and toward a large Chinese desk. On the desk was a book and scroll. Nigel told me the scroll was his, and he would go back to find it in China; it had messages for him.

He looked through the book, and as I watched him in this state, I saw a glow, an aura of peace and perfection. He told me this book was to be one of his next guides and the Chinese man to be one of his teachers. He asked to spend time in meditation and counsel with his teacher, as he had guidance to learn. I was overwhelmed by the sweet serenity of the occasion and felt honored to be present. I chose not to look further but remain at a respectful distance.

I sat silently and waited, allowing the meeting to take place. When it was finished, Nigel indicated that he was ready to leave. I guided him to the elevator, and we went back to the base level and returned to our world.

When the session was over he was delighted.

"You know," I said, "I saw a man I would describe as Confucius, a wise one, but I'm not sure."

He laughed and said, "Yes, he is my new teacher and had information for me, so we created focus and knowledge going forward."

A few weeks later, Nigel called me to tell me he had been helping his little old lady neighbor the previous day, and she had a Chinese nephew. When they spoke, he was told they were descendants of Confucius and had access to some of the ancient books. She told him should he wish, he could visit and connect with the wisdom and energy of this amazing man, wise beyond his time.

How divine.

What I find wonderful is that Akashic progression can help people locate the lessons of the future or the guides they will work with. The Akashic has given me the elevator or staircase method to help you reach into your future and how to redirect yourself back to other dimensions.

I will sometimes create the billboard message, a large sign, to illustrate words or messages to you. Those who are not visual may hear the word or feel the emotion. This projects high vibration frequencies of light into future time and lives.

Future or progression sessions are also a great way of imprinting positive intention and vibration forward in your lives. I must add at this point, however, that if you ask for peace but are manifesting and surrounding yourself with chaos, something has to shift, and it always starts with you.

This is my number-one rule: "Fit your own oxygen mask first, before helping others."

Future progression has helped many of my friends in this time of change. The energies around us are changing, and so are we. This challenges our egos and rational minds. I'm seeing competent, amazing people leave relationships, go bankrupt, yet still with a positive forward focus. They move forward and manifest greater joy and happiness in their lives.

Once you support yourself with your own vision and mission of soul purpose, you find everything else is just "fluff and stuff." If you are working on your own spiritual journey, then the roles, relationships, and jobs you perform are simply ways to teach or enhance this experience.

Future life progression can also create a call to action or stimulus. I've had clients who watched loved ones leave and themselves grow old without reaching their vision of life. This can sometimes be distressing, and the important question is not what happened but how we can rewrite it and manifest a beautiful life for all.

People often ask the question, does karma from this life move into the next life?

This I have found was true; many clients would recall the drama from a recent previous life now reacting in the current life. However, as the energy of the planet is changing, I am finding that karma does not wait. Karma returns currently in this lifetime to clear. Many teachers have indicated this is a final lifetime of incarnation for certain souls. They are finally moving off the "wheel of life." They call this the golden lifetime and reaching ascension. After this, I'm told, souls of this high frequency can return home to their energy field, soul group, or soul star.

One spiritually advanced client had worked for many years on his path to enlightenment. He had visited the sacred sites, read the books, and meditated on every meaning of life. I was honored to work with Bruce on his question of "future life and purpose."

CASE STUDY—BRUCE

The "case" that had the greatest impact on me was the journeywork that we did on Roatan. That journey opened me up to inter-dimensional travel at a level that I had not previously experienced, and also showed me an ability that I had no idea existed let alone was capable of performing.

In a way, the "case" shook me to the core and very much had me questioning the direction I was taking with my own journey. It was a little overwhelming to know the impact I could have on other beings. That journey helped me to gain a new perspective of what we are capable of as 'beings' and a glimpse into my own abilities as a being beyond this 3D world. After quite a bit of reflection, I am feeling more comfortable in re-opening that aspect of life's journey albeit with a great deal of care and compassion.

Future Lives Meditation

Find yourself a quiet space and have your journal ready.

Ensure you have a sacred energy around you that brings clarity and safety.

Take a few deep breaths and relax and begin the meditation.

Now we begin, to open your Akashic record book.

Relax and allow your attention to wander to your heart.
Imagine a bright light growing in your heart
and spreading throughout your body.
See the light move down you lower body and
down through your legs, through your feet, and
like tree roots, all the way into the earth.
See your roots of shining light reach
the crystal of Gaia and connect.
As you do, you see the crystal sparkle and the
light rise back up though the roots into your
feet, legs, and body, back to the heart.
See the light rise from your heart and move
through your throat into your head. Like a
fountain, allow it to move up through your head
into the sky and connect with a star above.
See the light move back to you until the pulse
remains in your heart and the light that surrounds
you is a column from sky to earth.
Now focus on your heart, and let's warm it awake.
Imagine it has a glowing star with five points.
To open all the points, allow the heart energy to flow and
focus on the happiest moments or people in your life.

Relax and smile, and let the happy
thoughts expand this heart chakra.
Send light around this star.
Feel your shoulders relax back, and
feel the peace around you.
Now see a small flame in the center of the star.
Allow yourself to flow into the flame.
This is the flame of transformation and transmutation;
it clears negativity and brings purification and clarity.
Warm yourself in the flame and smile.
Now look down and see a pearl, a beautiful,
translucent, and radiant pearl.
Hold it in your hand, gently send it love,
and be amazed at how beautiful it is.
This is your heart, beloved, your divine heart,
the perfect essence of yourself when
you were created as a star seed.
And this is now the place you can visit and ask your truth.
You are connected to the Earth and
universe and in your divine heart.
Now is the time to open your sacred Akashic record book.
Ask to go to the area of the future.
Ask that you be able to access the knowledge
and truth beyond the dimensions.
Imagine yourself back in your library room.
Are any of your guides with you?
See your book on the desk, and open it with
your left hand. See it glow with golden light.

Then see a doorway appear in the room
with golden light shining behind it.
Move toward this door.
Open the door gently and step forward.
When you feel ready, look across the
room and see the elevator.
Walk toward the elevator.
As you reach it, hold the space and see the button.
Reach with your left hand and press for service.
When the door opens, step in and observe
the number of floors to choose from.
See the number of the floor come into your
consciousness, and feel the doors close.
As you reach the floor, step out.
Look around you.
Is this a future life?
Is this a teaching ashram?
What does the environment look like?
Who is with you?
How do you feel?

What is happening?
What have you returned to this Akashic record
to heal, clear, and gain clarity with?

What action do you need to take?
What words or emotions do you
wish to leave in this space?
See your record book, and write these
words on a clean new page.

What high-vibration lesson do you need to
know and return back to this lifetime with?
Just keep breathing, and smile light
energy into your heart.
Send love into this story.
Allow your higher spirit guides to step
forward to help you with this.
Who are your new teachers?
Spend time here in silence and listen.
When ready to leave, see the elevator
doors again in front of you.
Go back through the door and press the first-
floor button with your right hand.
Stand back in your garden sanctuary.
See your guide and gatekeeper.
Smile and take time to rest.
Send love into this story.
When ready, see the door again in front of you.
Go back through the door.
Close the door.
Stand back in your library.
Close your Akashic record book.
See your guides.
When ready, return to your space, see the light
disconnect from above and below, and create
an amazing feeling of joy in your heart.
Ground yourself and know you have achieved
a healing, clearing, and clarity.
If tears flow, let them.
Relax and take time in this sacred heart space of love.

Now take a moment to write the key points from your experience.

- What did you see?
- Who was there with you?
- What did you learn and discover about yourself?
- What clarity did you gain?
- What did you find and discover about divine purpose?
- What intentions did you place into the future and your records?
- What lessons and teachers will step toward you in the future?

Ancient wisdom, hear my prayer.
Ancient masters, work by my side.
Sacred energy, run through me.
I understand wisdom once forgotten.
I am radiating the divine heart once lost.
I reflect balance, bliss, and beauty.
I walk with the gentle flow of the Nile.
All things are now creating miracles
in my life here and now.

PART FOUR

Take an Akashic Journey to Egypt

Take an Akashic Journey to Egypt

The Great Pyramid at Giza holds many ancient secrets and mysteries. Interestingly, most are only witnessed with the clairvoyant eye. Over the years, many people have seen amazing sights, which has reinforced their knowledge that there is a whole bigger picture around us and we are not the only life form.

The Great Pyramid is often referred to as a tomb, and at certain times, I'm sure people were buried in there. My other belief is that this was a star chamber (a room which allows you to transport into other dimensions of the universe); certain vents in the structure at the top align with key star systems such as Sirius. I often refer to Sirius as the checking star or hub (like a major airport).

So many people who have taken Akashic sessions feel a great connection with Sirius, even though they do not feel their energy belongs at home there.

Egypt was home to the original mystery schools of initiation. That is why many feel connected or interested. Many clients are searching to find the place they knew in a past life where they most connected with their spiritual teachings—where they knew the ancient wisdom and always worked from their heart and soul.

After many years of tour-leading and ceremony initiations, I have found that each key temple that lies upon the Nile River has a unique purpose and gift to give. When I speak to groups, I will often reunite them back to ancient Egypt on an energetic level. I take them on a chakra meditation to align their energy points gently to those along the Nile. The final destination is the King's Chamber in the Great Pyramid in Cairo.

The best way to experience these temples is obviously to

visit and stand in their sacred spaces. However, in this busy world, many people are unable. This is my way of helping souls link with their wisdom and Egyptian heritage.

When working with the Akashic records in Egypt, I meditate with the ancient god named Thoth. He is often depicted standing with book or scribe pencil in hand. He is an amazing wise energy and a great teacher. Thoth created many of the books of wisdom, such as the Emerald Tablets. I was working in Luxor Temple when I came across a statue to Ramses II; on the back was a clear vision of Thoth, and opposite him Seshat. Both deities where over six feet tall and facing each other; they both held the scribe pencil. I sat and meditated with them both and saw how these energies supported each other. Seshat was divine feminine, and with the star above her head, she channeled the information from the Akashic. Thoth, as divine masculine, translated and created the written texts. I invoke both when I am working for balance and clarity.

Many people are able to revisit the temples through the divine heart meditation and recover the sacred knowledge and magic they left behind lifetimes ago.

Egypt is the most powerful place for energy I personally know on the planet.

I would be honored to guide you on a magic-carpet meditation through this mystical land.

Akashic Meditation to Egypt

Create your sacred space.

Relax and play soft meditation music.

Have water, a pen and paper. Do not worry about recording too much of this journey. Do not concern yourself if you do not see the full sacred site. See and visualize the color and the words. This meditation is an initiation and introduction to the energy. Certain names and places will resonate more deeply than others. You can journey deeper using the other meditations in the book at your own pace.

Ensure you have a sacred energy around you that brings clarity and safety.

Take a few deep breaths and relax
and begin the meditation.
Now we begin, to open your Akashic
record book to Egypt.
Relax and allow your attention to wander to your heart.
Connect your light to the center of the earth and
your crown to the stars in heaven above.
Surround yourself with a bubble of light.
Ask the ancient ones support your path and
open doorways to understanding.
Step into your sacred library and see
your Akashic sacred book.
See the pages open and a clean fresh empty page appear.
See the word *Egypt* appear upon the page.

Now see a door in front of you and a
guide waiting to hold your hand.
Walk toward this door of choice.
As you reach it, hold the space and see the handle.
Reach with your left hand and open the door.
Walk through and see the golden sand
of the desert around you.

Start to feel and see the color red around you.
See yourself standing in front of the
majestic temple at Abu Simbel.
See Thoth and Seshat greet you with gifts.
Allow balance to attract safe abundance all around you.
Feel the energy rise in your root chakra.
How do you feel?
What is happening?
What have you returned to this Akashic record
to heal, clear, and gain clarity with?
What action do you need to take?
Just keep breathing and smile light energy into your heart.
Send love into this story.

Start to feel and see the color orange around you.
See yourself standing in front of the
beautiful temple at Philae.
The true temple of Isis and divine feminine.
Allow relationships of conscious love
and light to surround you.
Feel the energy rise in your sacral chakra.

How do you feel?
What is happening?
What have you returned to this Akashic record
to heal, clear, and gain clarity with?
What action do you need to take?
Just keep breathing and smile light energy into your heart.
Send love into this story.

Start to feel and see the color yellow around you.
See yourself standing in front of the
empowering temple at Edfu.
The temple of Horus and the divine masculine.
Allow your true self and purpose to
shine and radiate around you.
Feel the energy rise in your solar plexus chakra.
How do you feel?
What is happening?
What have you returned to this Akashic record
to heal, clear, and gain clarity with?
What action do you need to take?
Just keep breathing and smile light energy into your heart.
Send love into this story.

Start to feel and see the color green around you.
See yourself standing in front of the divine temples
of Abydos with Osiris and Dendara with Hathor.
The temples of sacred union and sacred knowledge.

Allow your divine heart to expand with
beauty, bliss, and balance.
Feel the energy rise in your heart chakra.
How do you feel?
What is happening?
What have you returned to this Akashic record
to heal, clear, and gain clarity with?
What action do you need to take?
Just keep breathing and smile light energy into your heart.
Send love into this story.

Start to feel and see the color blue around you.
See yourself standing in front of the temple at Luxor.
The temple created to the one true
source of energy, light, and truth.
Hear Sekmet the lioness goddess roar.
Allow your voice to resonate with
compassion and wisdom.
Feel the energy rise in your throat chakra.
How do you feel?
What is happening?
What have you returned to this Akashic record
to heal, clear, and gain clarity with?
What action do you need to take?
Just keep breathing and smile light energy into your heart.
Send love into this story.

Start to feel and see the color indigo around you.

See yourself standing in front of the
Sphinx temple on Giza plateau.
Allow the wisdom and clairvoyant sight to grow in
your third eye and the records you seek re-appear.
Feel the energy rise in your third eye chakra.
How do you feel?
What is happening?
What have you returned to this Akashic record
to heal, clear, and gain clarity with?
What action do you need to take?
Just keep breathing and smile light energy into your heart.
Send love into this story.

Start to feel and see the color violet around you.
See yourself standing in front of the
Great Pyramid on Giza plateau.
Allow your connection to rise to the stars
in the universe in total gratitude.
See the sacred symbols appear, see the
invisible become visible once more.
Feel the energy rise in your crown chakra.
How do you feel?
What is happening?
What have you returned to this Akashic record
to heal, clear, and gain clarity with?
What action do you need to take?
Just keep breathing and smile light energy into your heart.
Send love into this story.

Breathe the energy into your whole being, and relax
in this amazing space of gratitude and light.
Your journey is gently ending for now.
See your guide and gatekeeper.
Smile, and if you need to, take time to rest.

When ready, return to your space.
See the light disconnect from above and below and
create an amazing feeling of joy in your heart.
Ground yourself and know you have achieved
a healing, clearing, and clarity.
If tears flow, let them.
Relax and take time in this sacred heart space of love.

Take a moment just to relax and the energy to settle in your body.

Record your experience.

- What did you feel?
- What did you experience?
- What did you see?
- What did you learn?
- What was the overwhelming emotion?
- Did you see symbols or messages?
- Which color brought up reactions?

This meditation may be visited as often as you feel able. Be gentle with yourself and always in your heart.

I am love

I am joy

I am life

I am beauty

I am positive

I am awake

I am heart

I am divine

PART FIVE

Living from
the Heart

LIVING WITH CONSCIOUSNESS

Consciousness as a state of mind is challenging; however, operating from the heart is very easy.

Throughout this book, we have moved through the divine heart meditation to enable you to move along your Akashic path. This heart space and conscious filter on the world allows us to see that there is no separation between ourselves and the universe.

You are a constant creator of your story, a cultivator of your karma and responsible for all the dharma balance in life.

When you work with the Akashic records and the sacred messages, the illusions of life fade away. The life patterns and contracts that hold you back from your truth fall away. It is a lifelong journey with roller-coaster experiences, if you're looking for them. At first the stories and messages may not appear. But never doubt that the initiations have now moved into your energy field.

Your guides are walking silently with you until you give them a gentle voice.

The cords that no longer serve you are ready to disappear.

The bliss, beauty, and balance are placed for you in your future.

All is in divine order; you have taken the first step in having a conversation with your subconscious and Akashic record books. It may have been lifetimes since you last truly connected with them. Send these amazing aspects of yourself love and light every day, and watch the magic unfold.

Embracing Your Higher Purpose

We all have value and purpose on this planet, even when we look around and see those more or less fortunate than ourselves. We all have a role to play in this earthbound experience of life and initiations. Some souls elect to show shadows of sadness in life to teach others compassion. Some souls choose a path of conscious living to enlighten others. I have a great theory that many of today's leaders, mentors, and teachers were the students in past lives who never got to complete the initiations of life.

When we truly understand Akashic work, we see that all are equal and have led the rich lives and the poor lives; been the prince and the pauper.

We are simply moving through phases and patterns as before.

Akashic therapy allows you to act as a helicopter, seeing all the aspects of your abilities. It sets you free to make the choices that serve your growth and peace within yourself. Your intuition and heart will guide you to a purpose that celebrates exactly the lessons you came to Earth to learn.

Find your heart and truth, embrace your lessons, and learn with vitality for life. Akashic records simply hold physical and mental timelines, like the hardware of a computer. You hold the destiny of your records, the emotional and spiritual software. Run the programs that serve your highest life purpose, and fly high in the dimensions of universal life.

ACKNOWLEDGMENTS

For many lifetimes I have waited to bring forward this energy teaching and healing. I am in deepest gratitude to those on the earth plane and other dimensions who have shone their light and supported the journey toward a greater consciousness.

I am immensely thankful to those who travelled to Egypt and reminded me of my soul purpose and deep knowledge of ancient teachings. Thank you dear Hakim Awyan, Christine Barraclough and ever always and forever Isis.

To Ryan and Jordan Romania who support their father and I to achieve our dreams, we adore and treasure you both.

To my parents Robert and Rita Errington who created the safe home in number 33 which was always grounded allowing me opportunity to fly higher than I could imagine.

To Rhonda Fleming who gracefully helped me open my sacred heart and Kate Spencer who continued to teach me to reach the further dimensions keeping my heart open.

To Shannon Kring Buset for inspiring my writing and being a true soul sister.

To Steve Romania my dearest beloved for the patience and proof reading.

To Helena Jevons for always holding me in my truth and creating a reality of the Akashic doctor.

To Debbie Dixon and David Harper for believing I could write a spiritual message and Hay House for opening doors of opportunity to express this Akashic work.

And finally to Kate Mackinnon and Dr Wayne Dyer who allowed my work to walk its talk during the Sacred Journey to Assisi, Lourdes and Medjigore. This truly was a gift of miracles.

About the Author

Amanda Romania is an international healer, teacher of intuition, and Akashic reader. For the past decade, she has worked with indigenous elders and shamans in the realm of sacred site energy and ritual. Amanda has a master's degree in business from Durham University and a doctorate in metaphysics.

Amanda has a passion and purpose to support others on their spiritual journey. She uses her gifts to engage individuals and groups with their heart and essence. Amanda teaches how to understand universal energy and how to apply this to everyday life.

Amanda's experience with the Akashic records is extensive; she has performed sessions all over the world, teaching a simple "how-to experience" for others, to empower themselves and gain healing, clearing and clarity with all aspects of their soul journey.

Amanda lives with her husband and children in England and the United States of America.

www.amandaromania.com

CPSIA information can be obtained
at www.ICGtesting.com
Printed in the USA
FSOW03n1524300415
6834FS